# THE COMPREHENSIVE GUIDE TO HERBAL REMEDIES

## A TRADITIONAL HOLISTIC APPROACH TO AILMENTS AND WELLNESS

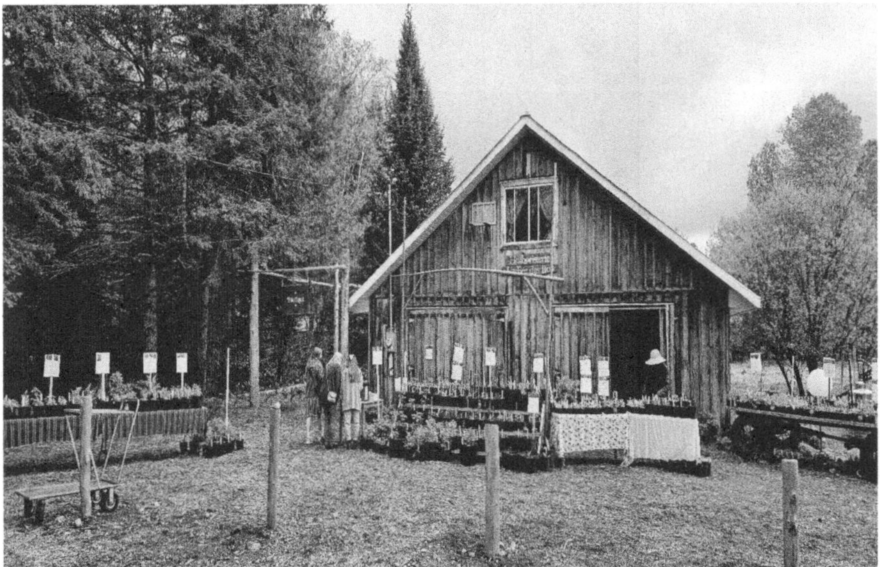

**Laurel Bennett**

# CONTENTS

# INTRODUCTION

## OVERVIEW OF HOLISTIC WELLNESS

In today's fast-paced world, many of us are seeking ways to take control of our health and well-being in a more natural, balanced way. Holistic wellness embraces the idea that health is not merely the absence of disease but the harmony of mind, body, and spirit. It is about nurturing all aspects of our lives—physical, emotional, mental, and even spiritual —using approaches that are in tune with nature.

Herbal remedies have been part of human wellness practices for thousands of years. In this book, we explore how herbs can support and enhance every aspect of your well-being, from the nourishment of your skin to the strengthening of your immune system. Whether you're looking to improve your hair care routine, soothe an upset stomach, or address more serious health concerns, herbs can offer a powerful, holistic solution.

By embracing the wisdom of plants and combining it with modern knowledge, herbal remedies help restore balance to the body. They are often gentle, safe, and supportive, acting in harmony with your body's natural rhythms. A holistic approach invites us to not only treat symptoms but to support overall wellness and vitality.

**Why Herbal Remedies?**

The use of herbs for medicinal and wellness purposes is as old as human history. From the ancient Egyptians and Chinese to Indigenous cultures across the world, plants have been the cornerstone of healing. Herbs provide a natural, effective way to manage many common health issues —whether you are looking to ease a sore throat, improve digestion, or manage stress. But the true power of herbal remedies lies in their ability to support the body's innate ability to heal itself.

Unlike synthetic medications, which can often provide quick relief with side effects, herbal remedies work gently with the body's systems to restore balance. Herbal medicine is founded on the understanding that plants contain compounds that nourish, support, and heal us, without the harshness of pharmaceuticals. For example, ginger, a well-known digestive aid, can soothe nausea and reduce inflammation, while chamomile offers gentle relaxation and stress relief.

However, herbs are not just a substitute for modern medicine. When used correctly, they can complement conventional treatments and provide a holistic, well-rounded approach to wellness. In this book, we'll dive into how to incorporate herbal remedies into your daily routine safely, whether you're using them for beauty care, to treat illness, or to enhance your overall health.

## HOW TO USE THIS BOOK

This book is designed to be both informative and practical, guiding you through the world of herbal remedies step by step. Each chapter provides insights into the most common herbs used for a particular purpose—whether it's for hair, skin, digestion, or immunity—and gives you the tools to make and apply these remedies in your own life.

You'll find:

• **Easy-to-follow herbal recipes**: Simple instructions to create teas, tinctures, oils, and balms at home.

• **Herb profiles**: Learn about each herb's benefits, how to use it, and where to find it.

• **Tips for safe use**: While herbs are natural, it's important to understand proper dosages and any potential side effects. We'll provide guidance on how to use herbs safely and effectively.

• **Holistic wellness tips**: In addition to herbs, we'll explore lifestyle practices, nutrition, and stress-management techniques to support your wellness journey.

As you journey through this book, remember that herbal remedies are not just about quick fixes—they're about embracing a lifestyle of wellness. Whether you are new to herbal medicine or an experienced practitioner, this guide will equip you with the knowledge and practical tools to nourish your body, mind, and spirit naturally.

So, get ready to explore the healing power of plants and transform your health through the wisdom of nature!

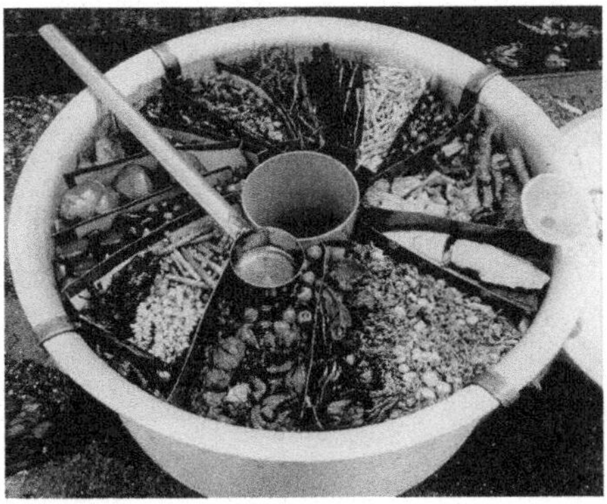

*Dried medicinal herbs*

# CHAPTER 1
# HERBAL COLD REMEDIES

Colds and respiratory issues are among the most common ailments we face, especially during colder months or when exposed to crowded environments. Understanding how colds spread, taking preventive measures, and using herbal remedies to alleviate symptoms can make a significant difference in recovery and overall wellness. This chapter explores herbal solutions for sore throats, flu relief, pneumonia support, coughs, and sinus issues, with practical recipes and tips for sourcing ingredients.

**Understanding How We Get Colds**

Colds are caused by viruses, primarily rhinoviruses, which spread through droplets in the air or via contact with contaminated surfaces. Once the virus enters the body through the nose, mouth, or eyes, it begins to replicate, triggering an immune response that leads to symptoms like sneezing, congestion, and sore throat.

**Preventing Colds**

- **Hand Hygiene:** Wash hands frequently with soap and water for at least 20 seconds. If soap and water are unavailable, use a hand sanitizer containing at least 60% alcohol.
- **Avoid Touching Your Face:** Reduce the likelihood of transferring viruses from your hands to your nose, mouth, or eyes.
- **Boost Your Immune System:** Maintain a healthy diet, get adequate sleep, and manage stress to keep your immune defenses strong.
- **Stay Hydrated:** Proper hydration helps maintain mucosal barriers in the respiratory tract, making it harder for viruses to take hold.

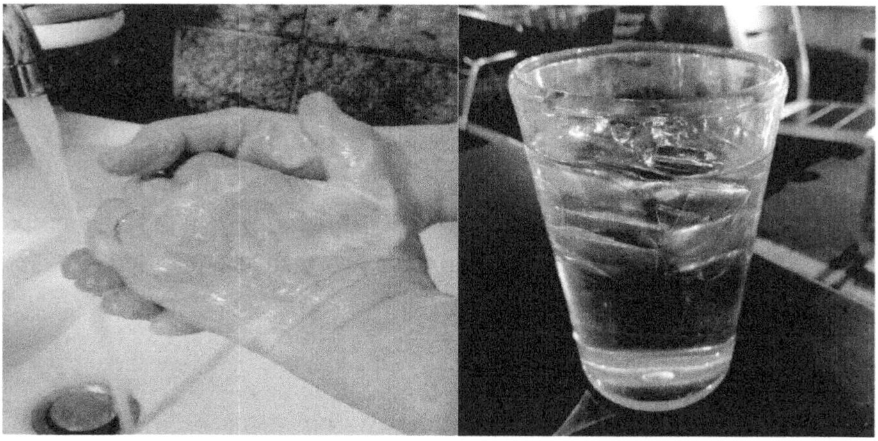

## PNEUMONIA SUPPORT

Pneumonia is a serious respiratory condition that often requires medical attention. Herbal remedies can complement medical treatments by supporting lung health, reducing inflammation, and easing breathing.

**Thyme Steam Inhalation**

Thyme helps loosen mucus and ease breathing.

*Ingredients*

- 1 tablespoon dried thyme
- 4 cups boiling water

*Instructions*

Add thyme to a bowl and pour boiling water over it.

Drape a towel over your head and the bowl to inhale the steam for 10 minutes.

*Where to Find Ingredients:* Thyme is available in grocery stores or herbal suppliers.

## HERBAL COUGH DROPS AND SYRUPS

Herbal cough remedies can soothe the throat and reduce coughing while promoting healing. Below are three recipes for herbal cough drops and three for herbal syrups.

**Herbal Cough Drops**

**Honey and Lemon Cough Drops**

*Ingredients*

- 1 cup raw honey
- Juice of 1 fresh lemon
- 1 teaspoon ground ginger

*Instructions*

In a saucepan, heat the honey, lemon juice, and ginger on low, stirring continuously until the mixture thickens.

Spoon small dollops onto parchment paper and let them cool and harden.

Store in an airtight container.

*Where to Find Ingredients:* Raw honey and lemons are available at grocery stores, and ground ginger can be found in the spice aisle.

**Eucalyptus and Mint Cough Drops**

*Ingredients*

- 1 cup sugar
- 1/2 cup water
- 10 drops eucalyptus essential oil
- 10 drops peppermint essential oil

*Instructions*

Combine sugar and water in a saucepan and heat until the sugar dissolves and forms a syrup.

Remove from heat and add the essential oils, stirring well.

Drop small amounts onto parchment paper and let harden.

*Where to Find Ingredients*: Essential oils are available in health food stores or online.

**Chamomile and Lavender Lozenges**

*Ingredients*

- 1/2 cup chamomile tea (brewed strongly)
- 1 cup honey
- 5 drops lavender essential oil

*Instructions*

Simmer honey and chamomile tea together until thickened.

Remove from heat and stir in lavender essential oil.

Pour into molds or drop small spoonfuls onto parchment paper and let cool.

*Where to Find Ingredients:* Chamomile tea and lavender essential oil can be found at herbal shops or online.

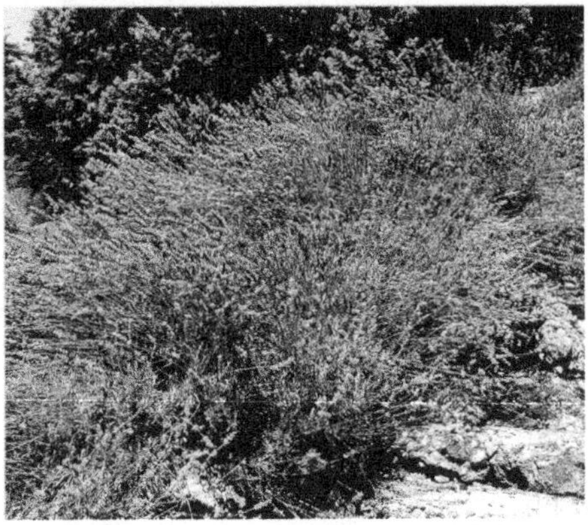

*Lavender*

## HERBAL SYRUPS

**Elderberry Syrup**

*Ingredients*

- 1 cup dried elderberries
- 4 cups water
- 1 cup raw honey

*Instructions*

Simmer elderberries in water for 30 minutes.

Strain and discard solids, then mix the liquid with raw honey.

Store in a sterilized bottle and take 1 tablespoon daily.

*Where to Find Ingredients*: Dried elderberries can be purchased from herbal suppliers or online.

**Thyme and Honey Syrup**

*Ingredients*

- 1/2 cup fresh thyme leaves
- 1 cup water
- 1 cup raw honey

*Instructions*

Boil thyme leaves in water for 10 minutes, then strain.

Mix the thyme-infused water with honey and heat gently until combined.

Store in a sterilized jar.

*Where to Find Ingredients*: Fresh thyme is available at grocery stores or farmer's markets.

**Ginger and Turmeric Syrup**

*Ingredients*

- 1-inch piece fresh ginger, grated
- 1/2 teaspoon ground turmeric
- 1 cup water
- 1 cup raw honey

*Instructions*

Simmer ginger and turmeric in water for 10 minutes, then strain.

Mix the strained liquid with honey and stir until smooth.

Store in a sterilized jar and take as needed.

*Where to Find Ingredients:* Ginger and turmeric are widely available in grocery stores.

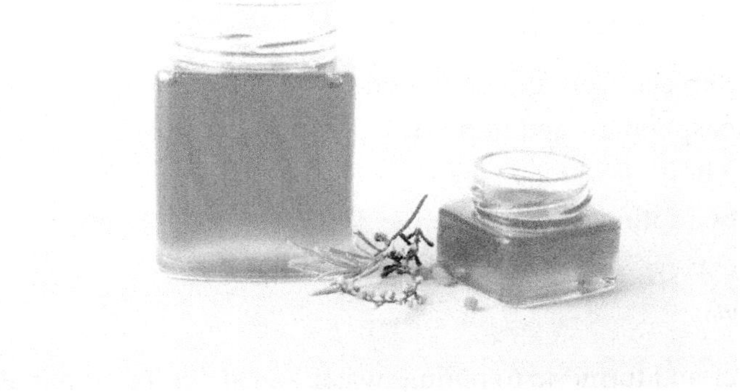

*Thyme and honey*

## HERBAL TEAS FOR SINUS ISSUES

Sinus congestion can be incredibly uncomfortable, leading to headaches and difficulty breathing. These herbal teas are designed to help reduce inflammation, promote drainage, and ease sinus pressure.

**Peppermint and Eucalyptus Tea**

*Ingredients*

- 1 teaspoon dried peppermint leaves
- 1 teaspoon eucalyptus leaves
- 1 cup boiling water

*Instructions*

Combine peppermint and eucalyptus leaves in a tea strainer.

Pour boiling water over the herbs and steep for 10 minutes.

Strain and sip slowly to relieve congestion.

*Where to Find Ingredients*: Dried peppermint leaves are available in herbal shops, and eucalyptus leaves can be found online or in specialty herb stores.

**Ginger and Turmeric Tea**

*Ingredients*

- 1-inch piece fresh ginger, sliced
- 1/2 teaspoon ground turmeric
- 1 cup boiling water
- Honey (optional)

*Instructions*

Add ginger and turmeric to boiling water and steep for 10 minutes.

Strain and sweeten with honey if desired.

Drink twice daily for sinus relief.

*Where to Find Ingredients:* Fresh ginger and ground turmeric are readily available in grocery stores.

**Chamomile and Thyme Tea**

*Ingredients*

- 1 tablespoon dried chamomile flowers
- 1 teaspoon dried thyme
- 1 cup boiling water

*Instructions*

Combine chamomile flowers and thyme in a tea strainer.

Steep in boiling water for 10 minutes.

Strain and sip warm.

*Where to Find Ingredients:* Chamomile flowers and dried thyme are available in herbal shops or online.

**Lemon Balm and Rosemary Tea**

*Ingredients*

- 1 teaspoon dried lemon balm leaves
- 1 teaspoon dried rosemary
- 1 cup boiling water

*Instructions*

Add lemon balm and rosemary to boiling water and steep for 10 minutes.

Strain and drink warm to ease sinus pressure.

*Where to Find Ingredients:* Both herbs can be purchased from herbal suppliers or health food stores.

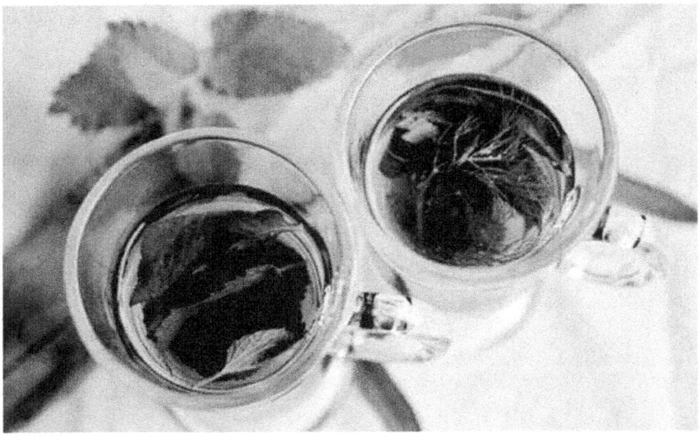

*Herbal teas*

**Spicy Cinnamon and Clove Tea**

*Ingredients*

- 1 cinnamon stick
- 3 whole cloves
- 1 cup boiling water

*Instructions*

Combine cinnamon and cloves in a tea strainer.

Steep in boiling water for 10 minutes.

Strain and sip to reduce congestion.

*Where to Find Ingredients:* Cinnamon sticks and cloves are widely available in the spice aisle of grocery stores.

CHAPTER 2

# HERBAL REMEDIES FOR UPSET STOMACH

Digestive issues can affect anyone, ranging from mild discomfort to more persistent conditions. Herbs have long been used to ease digestive discomfort, support overall gut health, and address specific ailments such as nausea, indigestion, and heartburn. In this chapter, we'll explore herbal solutions for these issues, including detailed recipes and guidance on sourcing the ingredients.

**Why We Experience Upset Stomachs**

Digestive discomfort can stem from various factors, including poor dietary habits, stress, food sensitivity, or underlying medical conditions. The digestive system is intricately connected to the rest of the body, and when it's not functioning optimally, it can lead to a range of symptoms such as bloating, gas, nausea, and cramps.

**Common Causes of Upset Stomachs:**

- **Dietary Choices:** Overeating, consuming processed foods, or eating too quickly can overwhelm the digestive system.
- **Stress:** Stress triggers the release of hormones that slow down digestion, leading to discomfort.

- **Food Intolerances:** Sensitivities to certain foods, like dairy or gluten, can cause bloating, gas, and other digestive issues.
- **Lack of Enzymes or Probiotics:** A healthy gut microbiome is essential for digestion. An imbalance in gut bacteria can lead to poor digestion and inflammation.
- **Dehydration:** Insufficient water intake can hinder digestion and cause constipation.
- **Underlying Conditions:** Issues such as gastroesophageal reflux disease (GERD), irritable bowel syndrome (IBS), or ulcers may contribute to chronic digestive discomfort.

**How to Maintain a Healthier Gut**

A healthy gut is essential for overall wellness, as it plays a vital role in nutrient absorption, immunity, and even mental health. Here are some ways to support and maintain a healthy digestive system:

**Eat a Balanced Diet**

- Focus on whole foods like fruits, vegetables, lean proteins, and whole grains.
- Include fiber-rich foods to promote regular bowel movements and prevent constipation.

**Stay Hydrated**

- Drink plenty of water throughout the day to support digestion and maintain the mucosal lining of the gut.

**Incorporate Probiotics**

- Probiotics are beneficial bacteria that support gut health. Foods like yogurt, kefir, sauerkraut, and kimchi are excellent sources.
- Consider a high-quality probiotic supplement if necessary.

**Manage Stress**

- Chronic stress can negatively impact the digestive system. Practice relaxation techniques such as deep breathing, yoga, or meditation.

**Chew Food Thoroughly**

- Digestion begins in the mouth. Chewing food thoroughly allows digestive enzymes to start breaking down food, reducing the workload on the stomach.

**Avoid Overeating**

- Eating smaller, more frequent meals can help prevent indigestion and bloating.

**Exercise Regularly**

- Physical activity stimulates intestinal movement, reducing the risk of constipation.

**Limit Processed Foods and Sugars**

- Excess sugar and processed foods can disrupt the balance of gut bacteria and lead to inflammation.

**Listen to Your Body**

- Identify and avoid trigger foods that cause discomfort.

**Use Herbal Remedies**

- Incorporating herbal teas, tinctures, and other remedies into your routine can support digestion and alleviate common digestive issues.

## DIGESTIVE HERBS

Herbs that support digestion often work by stimulating digestive enzymes, soothing inflammation, and reducing bloating. Below are common digestive herbs and their applications.

**Peppermint**

Peppermint is well-known for its ability to reduce bloating, cramping, and gas.

*How to Use*

- Brew as a tea or add fresh peppermint leaves to water.
- Use peppermint oil capsules for irritable bowel syndrome (IBS).

*Where to Find Ingredients:* Fresh peppermint leaves are available at grocery stores, while peppermint oil capsules can be purchased from pharmacies or online.

**Fennel**

Fennel seeds are excellent for reducing bloating and easing stomach cramps.

*How to Use*

- Chew on fennel seeds after meals.
- Brew as a tea by steeping 1 teaspoon of fennel seeds in boiling water.

*Where to Find Ingredients:* Fennel seeds are commonly available in the spice section of grocery stores.

**Ginger**

Ginger is a powerful anti-inflammatory and is particularly effective for nausea and motion sickness.

*How to Use*

- Add fresh ginger slices to hot water to make tea.
- Use powdered ginger in recipes or smoothies.

*Where to Find Ingredients:* Fresh ginger is widely available in grocery stores, and powdered ginger can be found in the spice aisle.

**Chamomile**

Chamomile is soothing for the digestive system and helps with bloating and mild cramping.

*How to Use*

- Brew chamomile tea by steeping 1 tablespoon of dried flowers in hot water.

*Where to Find Ingredients:* Chamomile flowers can be purchased from herbal suppliers or online.

**Dandelion Root**

Dandelion root supports liver function and helps stimulate digestion.

*How to Use*

- Use roasted dandelion root as a coffee substitute or brew it as tea.

*Where to Find Ingredients:* Dandelion root can be sourced from herbal shops or health food stores.

# CHAPTER 3
# EAR ACHE REMEDIES

Earaches are a common issue, affecting people of all ages. They can result from infections, fluid buildup, or inflammation in the ear canal. Herbal remedies can be a gentle and effective way to relieve pain, support ear health, and prevent recurring issues. This chapter explores herbs for ear health, provides step-by-step instructions for making herbal ear drops, and offers tips for preventing ear infections.

## HERBS FOR EAR HEALTH

Certain herbs are renowned for their antibacterial, antifungal, and anti-inflammatory properties, making them ideal for promoting ear health and alleviating pain.

### Garlic

Garlic is a powerful natural antibiotic and antifungal agent, making it highly effective against ear infections.

*How to Use*

- Infuse garlic in olive oil to create soothing ear drops.

*Where to Find Ingredients:* Fresh garlic is readily available in grocery stores, and olive oil can be found in any kitchen or supermarket.

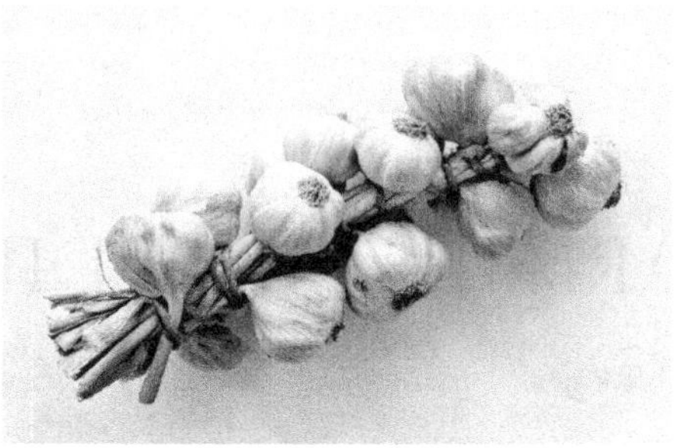

*Garlic*

**Mullein**

Mullein is well-known for its ability to soothe inflammation and reduce pain.

*How to Use*

- Use mullein-infused oil as an ear drop to calm irritation.

*Where to Find Ingredients:* Dried mullein flowers are available at herbal shops or online.

**Lavender**

Lavender has antimicrobial and anti-inflammatory properties, making it a gentle remedy for ear discomfort.

*How to Use*

- Combine lavender essential oil with a carrier oil for a soothing ear massage.

*Where to Find Ingredients:* Lavender essential oil can be purchased from health food stores or online retailers.

**Calendula**

Calendula is excellent for reducing inflammation and promoting healing.

*How to Use*

- Infuse calendula flowers in a carrier oil to create a gentle ear remedy.

*Where to Find Ingredients:* Dried calendula flowers can be sourced from herbal suppliers or health food stores.

**Tea Tree Oil**

Tea tree oil is a potent antimicrobial agent that can help fight infections.

*How to Use*

- Always dilute tea tree oil with a carrier oil before applying it near the ear.

*Where to Find Ingredients:* Tea tree oil is available at pharmacies, health food stores, and online.

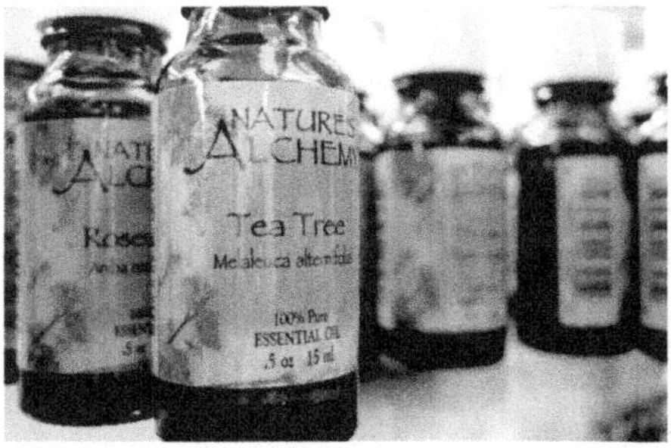


*Tea Tree Oil*

## HOW TO MAKE EAR DROPS

Homemade ear drops can provide relief from pain and discomfort while addressing the root cause of the problem. Below are some simple and effective recipes.

**Garlic and Olive Oil Ear Drops**

*Ingredients*

- 2 cloves fresh garlic
- 2 tablespoons olive oil

*Instructions*

Gently warm the olive oil in a small saucepan.

Crush the garlic cloves and add them to the oil.

Simmer on low heat for 10 minutes, then strain the oil to remove solids.

Let the oil cool to room temperature before using.

Apply 2-3 drops in the affected ear as needed.

*Where to Find Ingredients:* Fresh garlic and olive oil are widely available in grocery stores.

**Mullein and Calendula Ear Drops**

*Ingredients*

- 1 tablespoon dried mullein flowers
- 1 tablespoon dried calendula flowers
- 1/4 cup olive oil

*Instructions*

Place the dried flowers in a clean glass jar.

Cover with olive oil and seal tightly.

Allow the mixture to infuse for 2-4 weeks in a warm, dark place, shaking occasionally.

Strain the oil and store in a dropper bottle.

Use 2-3 drops in the ear as needed.

*Where to Find Ingredients:* Mullein and calendula flowers can be purchased from herbal suppliers or online.

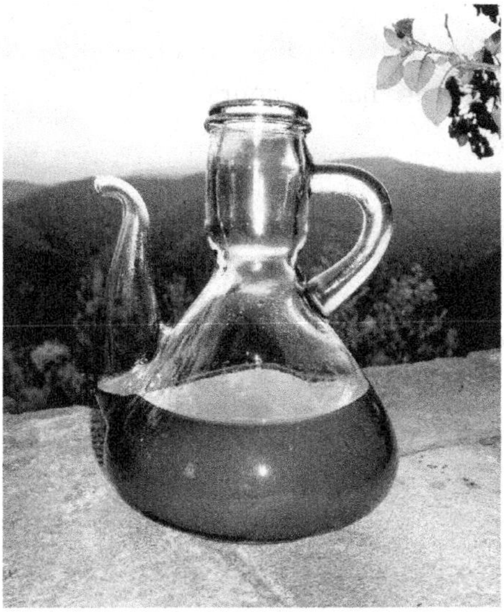

*Olive Oil*

**Tea Tree and Lavender Ear Oil**

*Ingredients*

- 1 tablespoon coconut oil
- 2 drops tea tree essential oil
- 2 drops lavender essential oil

*Instructions*

Melt the coconut oil in a small bowl.

Add tea tree and lavender essential oils and mix well.

Allow the oil to cool before use.

Apply 1-2 drops in the ear as needed.

*Where to Find Ingredients:* Coconut oil and essential oils are available at health food stores or online.

## PREVENTING EAR INFECTIONS

Preventing ear infections involves maintaining good hygiene and creating an environment that discourages bacterial or fungal growth. Here are some tips:

**Keep Ears Dry**

- After swimming or bathing, gently dry your ears with a towel or use ear-drying drops to prevent moisture buildup.

**Avoid Inserting Objects**

- Do not insert cotton swabs, fingers, or other objects into the ear canal, as this can introduce bacteria and cause irritation.

**Boost Your Immune System**

- A healthy immune system can reduce the risk of infections. Eat a balanced diet, stay hydrated, and get adequate sleep.

**Use Ear Protection**

- When swimming, consider using earplugs to prevent water from entering the ears.

**Address Allergies**

- Allergies can contribute to fluid buildup in the ears. Manage them with appropriate treatments to reduce the risk of infections.

**Avoid Smoking or Secondhand Smoke**

- Smoke can irritate the lining of the ears and make infections more likely.

**Practice Good Hygiene**

- Wash your hands regularly to reduce the spread of bacteria and viruses that could lead to ear infections.

# CHAPTER 4
# ALKALINE REMEDIES

Maintaining a balanced pH in the body is essential for overall health and vitality. Alkaline remedies, herbal teas, and an alkaline-focused diet can help support this balance, promoting wellness and preventing a range of health issues. In this chapter, we explore the concept of alkaline balance, herbal teas, and diet strategies, as well as recipes for herbal detox remedies.

## UNDERSTANDING ALKALINE BALANCE

Alkaline balance refers to the body's pH level, which measures how acidic or alkaline (basic) the internal environment is. The pH scale ranges from 0 to 14, with 7 being neutral. A pH below 7 indicates acidity, while a pH above 7 indicates alkalinity. The human body functions best at a slightly alkaline pH of around 7.35 to 7.45, particularly in the blood.

**Why Alkaline Balance Matters**

- **Health Optimization:** A balanced pH supports enzyme function, nutrient absorption, and cellular health.

- **Disease Prevention:** An overly acidic environment may contribute to chronic inflammation, fatigue, and diseases such as osteoporosis and kidney stones.
- **Energy Levels:** Maintaining alkalinity helps regulate energy production and reduce feelings of sluggishness.

### What Contributes to Acidity

- Consuming processed foods, sugar, and caffeine
- Stress and lack of sleep
- Environmental toxins

### How to Promote Alkalinity

- Incorporate more fresh fruits and vegetables into your diet.
- Stay hydrated with alkaline water or herbal teas.
- Practice stress management techniques such as yoga and deep breathing.

## HERBAL TEAS FOR ALKALINE BALANCE

Herbal teas can help restore the body's natural alkalinity by providing essential minerals and reducing acidity. Below are five recipes for herbal teas that support pH balance.

### Alfalfa and Nettle Tea

Alfalfa and nettle are rich in minerals that help alkalize the body.

*Ingredients*

- 1 teaspoon dried alfalfa leaves
- 1 teaspoon dried nettle leaves
- 1 cup boiling water

*Instructions*

Combine alfalfa and nettle in a tea strainer.

Pour boiling water over the herbs and steep for 10 minutes.

Strain and sip warm.

*Where to Find Ingredients:* Dried alfalfa and nettle leaves are available from herbal suppliers or online.

**Lemon Balm and Mint Tea**

This refreshing tea helps hydrate and alkalize the body.

*Ingredients*

- 1 teaspoon dried lemon balm leaves
- 1 teaspoon dried mint leaves
- 1 cup boiling water

*Instructions*

Steep lemon balm and mint in boiling water for 10 minutes.

Strain and enjoy warm or chilled.

*Where to Find Ingredients:* Dried lemon balm and mint leaves can be purchased from herbal shops or online.

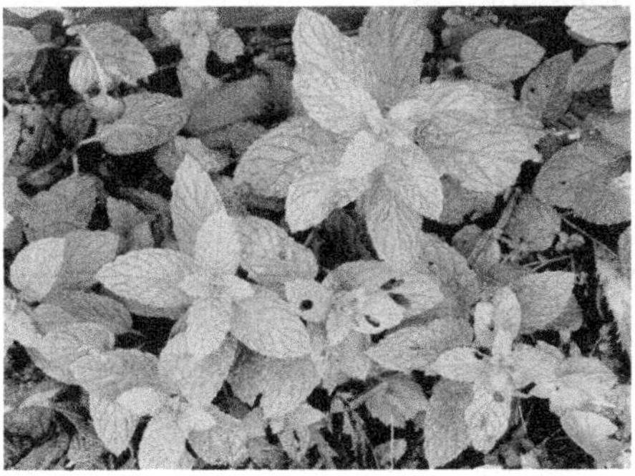

*Mint leaves*

**Chamomile and Dandelion Tea**

This tea combines chamomile's soothing properties with dandelion's alkalizing benefits.

*Ingredients*

- 1 tablespoon dried chamomile flowers
- 1 teaspoon dried dandelion root
- 1 cup boiling water

*Instructions*

Combine chamomile and dandelion in a tea strainer.

Pour boiling water over the herbs and steep for 10 minutes.

Strain and sip slowly.

*Where to Find Ingredients:* Chamomile flowers and dandelion root are widely available in health food stores or online.

**Parsley and Cilantro Detox Tea**

This tea supports alkalinity and detoxification.

*Ingredients*

- 1 tablespoon fresh parsley
- 1 tablespoon fresh cilantro
- 1 cup boiling water

*Instructions*

Chop parsley and cilantro and place them in a tea strainer.

Steep in boiling water for 10 minutes.

Strain and drink warm.

*Where to Find Ingredients:* Fresh parsley and cilantro are available at grocery stores or farmers' markets.

**Hibiscus and Rosehip Tea**

Rich in vitamin C, this tea helps reduce acidity and supports immune health.

*Ingredients*

- 1 teaspoon dried hibiscus petals
- 1 teaspoon dried rosehips
- 1 cup boiling water

*Instructions*

Steep hibiscus and rosehips in boiling water for 10 minutes.

Strain and serve warm or chilled.

*Where to Find Ingredients:* Dried hibiscus petals and rosehips can be sourced from herbal suppliers or online.

## ALKALINE DIET AND HERBS

A diet rich in alkaline-forming foods and herbs can help restore pH balance and promote overall health. Below are key strategies and recommendations:

**Focus on Alkaline-Forming Foods**

- Leafy greens like kale, spinach, and Swiss chard
- Fresh fruits, especially citrus, watermelon, and berries
- Root vegetables such as carrots and beets
- Nuts and seeds like almonds and flaxseeds

**Incorporate Alkalizing Herbs**

- Parsley, cilantro, and basil are excellent choices for cooking or making herbal teas.
- Use dried herbs like oregano and thyme for seasoning.

**Minimize Acid-Forming Foods**

- Limit red meat, processed foods, and sugary beverages.

**Stay Hydrated**

- Drink plenty of water, herbal teas, and fresh vegetable juices.

## HERBAL DETOX

Detoxification can help eliminate toxins that contribute to acidity. Below are five recipes for herbal detox remedies that promote alkalinity.

**Dandelion and Burdock Root Detox Tea**

*Ingredients*

- 1 teaspoon dried dandelion root
- 1 teaspoon dried burdock root
- 1 cup boiling water

*Instructions*

Combine dandelion and burdock root in a tea strainer.

Steep in boiling water for 10 minutes.

Strain and sip warm.

*Where to Find Ingredients:* Dandelion and burdock roots can be purchased from herbal shops or online.

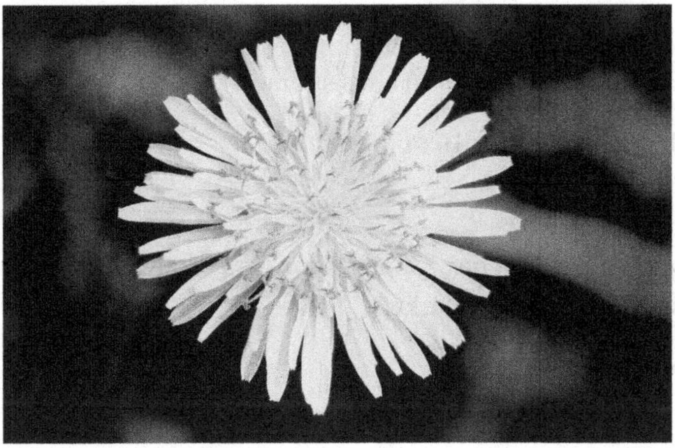

*Dandelion*

**Parsley and Lemon Juice Elixir**

*Ingredients*

- 1/4 cup fresh parsley, chopped
- Juice of 1 fresh lemon
- 1 cup warm water

*Instructions*

Blend parsley with lemon juice and warm water.

Strain if desired and drink immediately.

*Where to Find Ingredients:* Fresh parsley and lemons are available at grocery stores.

**Cilantro and Ginger Detox Infusion**

*Ingredients*

- 1 tablespoon fresh cilantro, chopped
- 1-inch piece fresh ginger, sliced
- 1 cup boiling water

*Instructions*

Combine cilantro and ginger in a tea strainer.

Steep in boiling water for 10 minutes.

Strain and drink warm.

*Where to Find Ingredients:* Cilantro and ginger are widely available at grocery stores or farmers' markets.

**Green Smoothie Detox**

*Ingredients*

- 1 cup spinach leaves
- 1/2 cucumber, sliced
- Juice of 1 lime
- 1 cup water

*Instructions*

Blend all ingredients until smooth.

Drink immediately for a refreshing detox boost.

*Where to Find Ingredients:* Spinach, cucumber, and lime are available in grocery stores or farmers' markets.

**Basil and Mint Detox Water**

*Ingredients*

- 1/4 cup fresh basil leaves
- 1/4 cup fresh mint leaves
- 1 liter water

*Instructions*

Add basil and mint leaves to a pitcher of water.

Let infuse for 2-4 hours in the refrigerator.

Drink throughout the day.

*Where to Find Ingredients:* Fresh basil and mint can be purchased at grocery stores or farmers' markets.

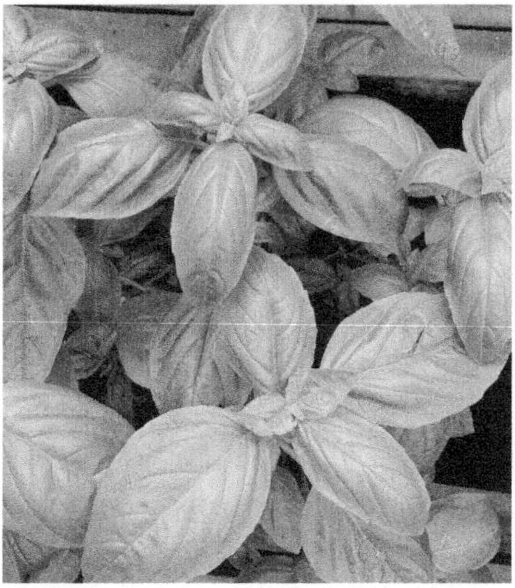

*Basil*

CHAPTER 5

# RHEUMATOID ARTHRITIS RELIEF AND MANAGEMENT

Rheumatoid arthritis (RA) is an autoimmune condition that causes chronic inflammation, joint pain, and stiffness. Managing RA naturally involves reducing inflammation, supporting joint health, and easing pain through diet, lifestyle changes, and herbal remedies. This chapter explores effective herbal solutions to alleviate symptoms and improve overall mobility. Whether you're looking for pain relief, inflammation reduction, or improved joint function, these natural remedies will support your wellness journey.

## REDUCING INFLAMMATION

Chronic inflammation is the main contributor to RA symptoms. These herbal remedies help combat inflammation and support immune function.

**Turmeric and Ginger Anti-Inflammatory Tonic**

*Ingredients*

- 1 teaspoon ground turmeric
- 1 teaspoon grated fresh ginger

- 1 cup warm almond or coconut milk
- 1 teaspoon raw honey (optional)

*Instructions*

Mix turmeric and ginger into warm milk.

Sweeten with honey if desired.

Drink daily to reduce inflammation and joint pain.

*Where to Find Ingredients:* Turmeric and ginger are widely available in grocery stores.

**Boswellia and Clove Joint Support Tea**

*Ingredients*

- 1 teaspoon dried boswellia (Indian frankincense)
- 1/2 teaspoon ground clove
- 1 cup boiling water

*Instructions*

Steep boswellia and clove in boiling water for 10 minutes.

Strain and sip slowly to relieve inflammation.

*Where to Find Ingredients:* Boswellia and clove can be found in herbal shops or online.

**Rosemary and Green Tea Anti-Inflammatory Infusion**

*Ingredients*

- 1 teaspoon dried rosemary
- 1 teaspoon green tea leaves
- 1 cup boiling water

*Instructions*

Steep rosemary and green tea in boiling water for 10 minutes.

Strain and enjoy to support joint function and immune health.

*Where to Find Ingredients:* Both ingredients are available in grocery stores and herbal shops.

**Licorice Root and Cinnamon Soothing Tea**

*Ingredients*

- 1 teaspoon dried licorice root
- 1/2 teaspoon ground cinnamon
- 1 cup boiling water

*Instructions*

Steep licorice root and cinnamon in boiling water for 10 minutes.

Strain and sip warm for relief from inflammation.

*Where to Find Ingredients:* Herbal suppliers and online retailers carry these dried herbs.

**Flaxseed and Chia Omega-3 Booster**

*Ingredients*

- 1 teaspoon ground flaxseed
- 1 teaspoon chia seeds
- 1 cup warm water

*Instructions*

Stir flaxseed and chia seeds into warm water.

Let sit for 10 minutes before drinking.

Consume daily to support joint lubrication and reduce inflammation.

*Where to Find Ingredients:* Grocery stores and health food stores carry flaxseed and chia seeds.

## PAIN AND STIFFNESS RELIEF

Joint pain and stiffness are common RA symptoms. These herbal remedies help relieve discomfort and promote better movement.

**Willow Bark and Chamomile Pain-Relief Tea**

*Ingredients*

- 1 teaspoon dried willow bark
- 1 teaspoon dried chamomile flowers
- 1 cup boiling water

*Instructions*

Steep willow bark and chamomile in boiling water for 15 minutes.

Strain and sip to ease joint pain.

*Where to Find Ingredients:* Herbal suppliers and online retailers carry these dried herbs.

**Peppermint and Eucalyptus Joint Soothing Rub**

*Ingredients*

- 2 tablespoons coconut oil
- 5 drops peppermint essential oil
- 5 drops eucalyptus essential oil

*Instructions*

Mix oils together and apply to sore joints.

Massage gently for relief.

*Where to Find Ingredients:* Essential oils are available at health food stores and online.

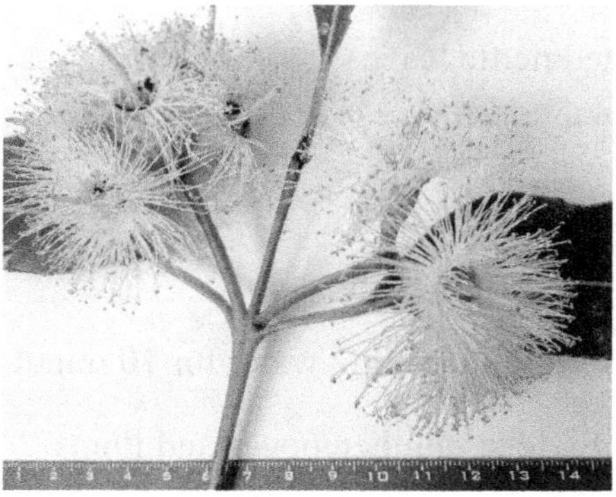

*Eucalyptus flowers*

**Epsom Salt and Lavender Bath Soak**

*Ingredients*

- 1/2 cup Epsom salt
- 5 drops lavender essential oil
- Warm bathwater

*Instructions*

Dissolve Epsom salt in warm bathwater.

Add lavender essential oil and soak for 20 minutes.

Repeat as needed for pain relief.

*Where to Find Ingredients:* Epsom salt is available at pharmacies, and lavender oil can be found in herbal shops.

## SUPPORTING JOINT HEALTH

Maintaining joint mobility and health is crucial for RA management. These herbal remedies support flexibility and strengthen joints.

**Nettle and Horsetail Bone Strengthening Tea**

*Ingredients*

- 1 teaspoon dried nettle leaves
- 1 teaspoon dried horsetail
- 1 cup boiling water

*Instructions*

Steep nettle and horsetail in boiling water for 10 minutes.

Strain and drink daily to strengthen bones and joints.

*Where to Find Ingredients:* Herbal suppliers and online retailers carry these dried herbs.

**Alfalfa and Turmeric Joint Nourishing Infusion**

*Ingredients*

- 1 teaspoon dried alfalfa leaves
- 1/2 teaspoon ground turmeric
- 1 cup boiling water

*Instructions*

Steep alfalfa and turmeric in boiling water for 10 minutes.

Strain and drink to support joint health.

*Where to Find Ingredients:* Dried herbs can be purchased from herbal suppliers or online.

Rheumatoid arthritis can be challenging, but with the right natural remedies, you can manage symptoms and improve mobility. These herbal solutions help reduce inflammation, ease joint pain, and support long-term joint health, giving you the tools to take control of your well-being naturally.

# CHAPTER 6
# GENERAL WELLNESS

Maintaining overall wellness requires a balanced approach that nurtures the mind, body, and spirit. By focusing on natural ways to boost immunity, manage stress, enhance energy, support restful sleep, and improve mental clarity, you can create a foundation for lasting health. This chapter explores herbs and practices that target these areas, with practical recipes and strategies for integrating them into your daily routine. Whether you're looking to ward off seasonal illnesses, handle stress with more ease, or simply feel more energized and focused, the remedies in this chapter are designed to empower your wellness journey.

## BOOSTING IMMUNITY

A strong immune system is your body's best defense against infections and illnesses. Below are five herbal recipes to help strengthen immunity naturally.

**Elderberry and Echinacea Immune Syrup**

*Ingredients*

- 1 cup dried elderberries
- 1/2 cup dried echinacea root
- 4 cups water
- 1 cup raw honey

*Instructions*

Combine elderberries, echinacea root, and water in a saucepan.

Simmer on low heat for 30 minutes.

Strain and discard solids, then stir in raw honey while the liquid is warm.

Store in a sterilized jar and take 1 tablespoon daily as a preventive measure.

*Where to Find Ingredients:* Dried elderberries and echinacea root can be purchased from herbal suppliers or online.

**Garlic and Lemon Immune Tonic**

*Ingredients*

- 3 cloves fresh garlic, minced
- Juice of 1 fresh lemon
- 1 tablespoon raw honey
- 1 cup warm water

*Instructions*

Mix garlic, lemon juice, and honey into warm water.

Let it steep for 10 minutes.

Drink once daily to support immune function.

*Where to Find Ingredients:* Fresh garlic and lemons are available at grocery stores, and raw honey can be found in health food stores.

**Turmeric and Ginger Immunity Tea**

*Ingredients*

- 1-inch piece fresh ginger, sliced
- 1/2 teaspoon ground turmeric
- 1 cup boiling water
- Honey (optional)

*Instructions*

Add ginger and turmeric to boiling water.

Steep for 10 minutes, then strain.

Sweeten with honey if desired.

*Where to Find Ingredients:* Fresh ginger and ground turmeric are widely available in grocery stores.

**Astragalus and Rosehip Infusion**

*Ingredients*

- 1 tablespoon dried astragalus root
- 1 tablespoon dried rosehips
- 1 cup boiling water

*Instructions*

Steep astragalus root and rosehips in boiling water for 15 minutes.

Strain and drink warm.

*Where to Find Ingredients:* Dried astragalus root and rosehips can be purchased from herbal shops or online.

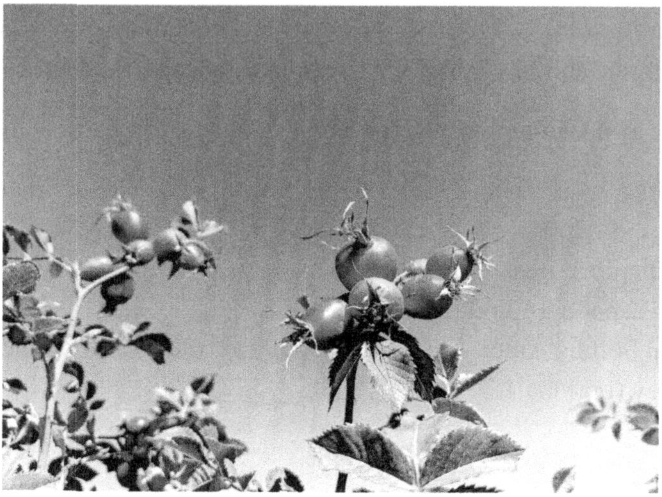

*Rosehips*

**Vitamin C-Rich Citrus Elixir**

*Ingredients*

- Juice of 1 orange
- Juice of 1 lemon
- 1 teaspoon grated ginger
- 1 teaspoon raw honey

*Instructions*

Mix orange juice, lemon juice, ginger, and honey in a glass.

Stir well and drink immediately.

*Where to Find Ingredients:* Citrus fruits and ginger are available in grocery stores, and raw honey can be found at health food stores.

## STRESS REDUCTION AND ADAPTOGENS

Adaptogens are herbs that help the body adapt to stress and restore balance. Below are recipes to help you manage stress naturally.

**Ashwagandha and Cinnamon Latte**

*Ingredients*

- 1 teaspoon ashwagandha powder
- 1/2 teaspoon ground cinnamon
- 1 cup warm almond milk
- 1 teaspoon raw honey

*Instructions*

Mix ashwagandha powder and cinnamon into warm almond milk.

Sweeten with honey and enjoy before bedtime.

*Where to Find Ingredients:* Ashwagandha powder and ground cinnamon are available in health food stores or online.

**Holy Basil Tea**

*Ingredients*

- 1 teaspoon dried holy basil (tulsi)
- 1 cup boiling water

*Instructions*

Steep holy basil in boiling water for 10 minutes.

Strain and drink warm to promote relaxation.

*Where to Find Ingredients:* Holy basil can be found in herbal shops or online.

**Lavender and Chamomile Stress Tea**

*Ingredients*

- 1 teaspoon dried lavender flowers
- 1 teaspoon dried chamomile flowers

- 1 cup boiling water

*Instructions*

Combine lavender and chamomile in a tea strainer.

Pour boiling water over the herbs and steep for 10 minutes.

Strain and sip slowly.

*Where to Find Ingredients:* Dried lavender and chamomile flowers are available in herbal shops or online.

**Rhodiola Rosea Elixir**

*Ingredients*

- 1 teaspoon rhodiola rosea powder
- 1 cup warm water
- 1 teaspoon honey (optional)

*Instructions*

Mix rhodiola powder into warm water.

Sweeten with honey if desired.

Drink in the morning to enhance focus and resilience.

*Where to Find Ingredients:* Rhodiola powder is available at health food stores or online.

**Lemon Balm and Peppermint Infusion**

*Ingredients*

- 1 teaspoon dried lemon balm
- 1 teaspoon dried peppermint
- 1 cup boiling water

*Instructions*

Steep lemon balm and peppermint in boiling water for 10 minutes.

Strain and enjoy warm.

*Where to Find Ingredients:* Both herbs can be found at herbal suppliers or online.

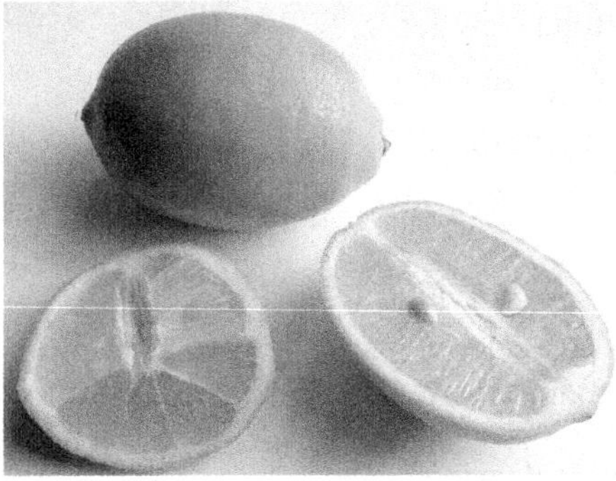

*Lemons*

## ENERGY-BOOSTING HERBS

Herbs can provide a natural and sustained energy boost without the jittery effects of caffeine. Below are recipes to enhance vitality and endurance.

**Ginseng and Ginger Energy Tea**

*Ingredients*

- 1 teaspoon dried ginseng root
- 1 teaspoon fresh ginger, sliced
- 1 cup boiling water

*Instructions*

Combine ginseng root and ginger in a tea strainer.

Steep in boiling water for 15 minutes.

Strain and sip to boost energy levels.

*Where to Find Ingredients:* Dried ginseng root is available in herbal shops, and fresh ginger can be purchased at grocery stores.

**Matcha and Maca Latte**

*Ingredients*

- 1 teaspoon matcha powder
- 1 teaspoon maca powder
- 1 cup warm almond milk
- 1 teaspoon honey (optional)

*Instructions*

Whisk matcha and maca powders into warm almond milk.

Sweeten with honey if desired.

Drink in the morning for sustained energy.

*Where to Find Ingredients:* Matcha and maca powders can be found in health food stores or online.

**Rosemary and Lemon Energy Infusion**

*Ingredients*

- 1 teaspoon dried rosemary
- Juice of 1/2 lemon
- 1 cup boiling water

*Instructions*

Steep rosemary in boiling water for 10 minutes.

Add lemon juice and drink warm.

*Where to Find Ingredients:* Dried rosemary is available in the spice aisle, and lemons can be purchased at grocery stores.

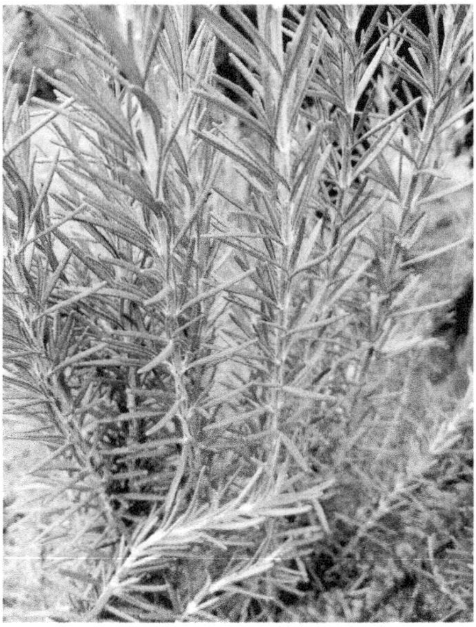

*Rosemary*

**Eleuthero Root Tonic**

*Ingredients*

- 1 teaspoon dried eleuthero root
- 1 cup boiling water

*Instructions*

Steep eleuthero root in boiling water for 15 minutes.

Strain and drink to support endurance and energy.

*Where to Find Ingredients:* Eleuthero root can be purchased from herbal suppliers or online.

**Peppermint and Licorice Energy Tea**

*Ingredients*

- 1 teaspoon dried peppermint leaves

- 1 teaspoon dried licorice root
- 1 cup boiling water

*Instructions*

Steep peppermint and licorice root in boiling water for 10 minutes.

Strain and enjoy warm.

*Where to Find Ingredients:* Both ingredients are available in herbal shops or online.

## SLEEP SUPPORT

Sleep is essential for physical and mental health, and herbs can help promote relaxation and improve sleep quality. Below are herbal recipes to support restful sleep.

**Chamomile and Lavender Sleep Tea**

*Ingredients*

- 1 tablespoon dried chamomile flowers
- 1 teaspoon dried lavender flowers
- 1 cup boiling water

*Instructions*

Combine chamomile and lavender in a tea strainer.

Pour boiling water over the herbs and steep for 10 minutes.

Strain and sip slowly before bedtime.

*Where to Find Ingredients:* Dried chamomile and lavender flowers are available in herbal shops or online.

**Valerian Root Bedtime Tonic**

*Ingredients*

- 1 teaspoon dried valerian root
- 1 cup boiling water

*Instructions*

Steep valerian root in boiling water for 10-15 minutes.

Strain and drink 30 minutes before bed.

*Where to Find Ingredients:* Dried valerian root can be found at herbal suppliers or online.

**Passionflower and Lemon Balm Sleep Tea**

*Ingredients*

- 1 teaspoon dried passionflower
- 1 teaspoon dried lemon balm
- 1 cup boiling water

*Instructions*

Combine passionflower and lemon balm in a tea strainer.

Steep in boiling water for 10 minutes.

Strain and drink to calm the mind.

*Where to Find Ingredients:* Both herbs are available at herbal suppliers or online.

**Hops and Honey Relaxation Tea**

*Ingredients*

- 1 teaspoon dried hops flowers
- 1 teaspoon honey

- 1 cup boiling water

*Instructions*

1. Steep hops flowers in boiling water for 10 minutes.
2. Strain and stir in honey before drinking.

*Where to Find Ingredients:* Dried hops flowers are available at herbal shops or online.

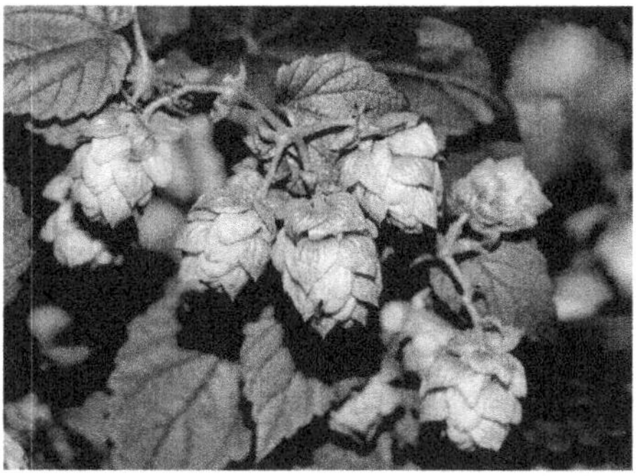

*Hops*

## HERBS FOR MENTAL CLARITY

Mental clarity is essential for focus, productivity, and overall well-being. Below are herbal recipes to enhance cognitive function.

**Rosemary and Sage Brain Boost Tea**

*Ingredients*

- 1 teaspoon dried rosemary
- 1 teaspoon dried sage
- 1 cup boiling water

*Instructions*

Combine rosemary and sage in a tea strainer.

Steep in boiling water for 10 minutes.

Strain and drink to improve concentration.

*Where to Find Ingredients:* Dried rosemary and sage can be purchased in the spice aisle or herbal shops.

**Ginkgo Biloba and Peppermint Tea**

*Ingredients*

- 1 teaspoon dried ginkgo biloba leaves
- 1 teaspoon dried peppermint
- 1 cup boiling water

*Instructions*

Steep ginkgo biloba and peppermint in boiling water for 10 minutes.

Strain and enjoy warm.

*Where to Find Ingredients:* Dried ginkgo biloba and peppermint are available from herbal suppliers.

**Gotu Kola and Lemon Balm Focus Tea**

*Ingredients*

- 1 teaspoon dried gotu kola
- 1 teaspoon dried lemon balm
- 1 cup boiling water

*Instructions*

Combine gotu kola and lemon balm in a tea strainer.

Steep in boiling water for 10 minutes.

Strain and sip warm to enhance focus.

*Where to Find Ingredients:* Gotu kola and lemon balm are available at herbal shops or online.

**Tulsi and Cinnamon Mental Clarity Tea**

*Ingredients*

- 1 teaspoon dried tulsi (holy basil)
- 1/2 teaspoon ground cinnamon
- 1 cup boiling water

*Instructions*

Steep tulsi and cinnamon in boiling water for 10 minutes.

Strain and enjoy warm for a mental boost.

*Where to Find Ingredients:* Tulsi and cinnamon are widely available in herbal shops and grocery stores.

**Lion's Mane and Ginger Elixir**

*Ingredients*

- 1 teaspoon lion's mane mushroom powder
- 1 teaspoon grated fresh ginger
- 1 cup boiling water

*Instructions*

Mix lion's mane powder and ginger in a cup.

Pour boiling water over the mixture and stir well.

Drink to support cognitive function.

*Where to Find Ingredients:* Lion's mane powder and fresh ginger are available at health food stores and online.

CHAPTER 7

# HERBS AND SPICES FOR NUTRITION

Incorporating herbs and spices into your diet is a simple and effective way to enhance your overall nutrition. Many herbs and spices not only add flavor but also provide essential vitamins, minerals, and antioxidants that promote health and prevent disease. In this chapter, we will explore nutritional herbs, healing spices, tips for incorporating them into your daily meals, and guidelines for using herbal supplements and powders safely and effectively.

## NUTRITIONAL HERBS

Herbs are packed with nutrients and bioactive compounds that support overall wellness. Below are some common nutritional herbs, their benefits, and tips cues to help you use them with confidence.

**Parsley**

- **Benefits:** High in vitamin K, C, and iron, parsley supports bone health and boosts immunity.
- **Usage:** Add fresh parsley to soups, salads, and smoothies.

**Nettle**

- **Benefits:** Rich in calcium, magnesium, and iron, nettle promotes bone strength and energy levels.
- **Usage:** Brew as tea or use dried nettle in soups and stews.

**Dandelion**

- **Benefits:** Supports liver health and digestion, and is high in vitamin A and potassium.
- **Usage:** Use dandelion greens in salads or brew the root into a tea.

**Basil**

- **Benefits:** Contains vitamin A, K, and manganese; supports heart health and reduces inflammation.
- **Usage:** Add fresh basil to pasta, sandwiches, and sauces.

**Oregano**

- **Benefits:** A powerful antioxidant, oregano supports immune health and digestion.
- **Usage:** Sprinkle dried oregano over roasted vegetables or pizza.

**Thyme**

- **Benefits:** Antibacterial and rich in vitamins C and A, thyme supports respiratory and immune health.
- **Usage:** Add to soups, marinades, and roasted meats.

**Chamomile**

- **Benefits:** Calming properties help reduce stress and support sleep.

- **Usage:** Brew as tea or use in desserts and infused syrups.

**Lemon Balm**

- **Benefits:** Reduces anxiety, improves sleep, and supports digestion.
- **Usage:** Add to teas, desserts, or infused waters.

**Sage**

- **Benefits:** Contains anti-inflammatory compounds and supports memory and focus.
- **Usage:** Use fresh or dried in stuffing, sauces, or teas.

**Rosemary**

- **Benefits:** Improves memory, circulation, and digestion.
- **Usage:** Infuse in oils, add to roasted vegetables, or brew as tea.

**Lavender**

- **Benefits:** Promotes relaxation and reduces anxiety.
- **Usage:** Use dried flowers in teas, desserts, or infused sugars.

**Mullein**

- **Benefits:** Supports respiratory health and soothes inflammation.
- **Usage:** Brew as tea or infuse in oils for topical use.

**Holy Basil**

- **Benefits:** Adaptogen that helps reduce stress and improve focus.
- **Usage:** Brew as tea or use fresh leaves in curries and stir-fries.

**Cilantro**

- **Benefits:** Supports detoxification and is rich in antioxidants.
- **Usage:** Add fresh to salsas, salads, and soups.

**Peppermint**

- **Benefits:** Eases digestion and reduces headaches.
- **Usage:** Brew as tea or add fresh leaves to drinks and desserts.

## SPICES THAT HEAL

Spices not only enhance flavor but also offer medicinal properties. Here are some healing spices with their benefits and usage.

**Turmeric**

- **Benefits:** Contains curcumin, a potent anti-inflammatory and antioxidant.
- **Usage:** Add to curries, golden milk, or rice dishes.

**Cinnamon**

- **Benefits:** Helps regulate blood sugar and has antibacterial properties.
- **Usage:** Sprinkle on oatmeal, yogurt, or coffee.

**Ginger**

- **Benefits:** Aids digestion, reduces nausea, and has anti-inflammatory effects.
- **Usage:** Add fresh ginger to tea, stir-fries, or smoothies.

**Clove**

- **Benefits:** Contains eugenol, which supports oral health and digestion.
- **Usage:** Use in spice blends, baked goods, or mulled beverages.

**Cayenne Pepper**

- **Benefits:** Boosts metabolism and supports circulation.
- **Usage:** Sprinkle on eggs, avocado toast, or roasted vegetables.

**Nutmeg**

- **Benefits:** Contains compounds that support digestion and relaxation.
- **Usage:** Grate fresh nutmeg into sauces, baked goods, and beverages.

**Cardamom**

- **Benefits:** Supports digestion and respiratory health.
- **Usage:** Add to curries, teas, or desserts.

**Black Pepper**

- **Benefits:** Enhances nutrient absorption and supports digestion.
- **Usage:** Use in spice blends or sprinkle freshly ground over meals.

**Fennel Seed**

- **Benefits:** Reduces bloating and improves digestion.
- **Usage:** Chew raw seeds or use in teas and spice blends.

**Anise**

- **Benefits:** Supports digestion and reduces nausea.
- **Usage:** Add to teas, baked goods, or stews.

## HOW TO INCORPORATE HERBS INTO YOUR DIET

Incorporating herbs into your diet is easy and rewarding. Start by using fresh herbs as garnishes for salads, soups, and main dishes. Dried herbs can be added to spice blends, marinades, or baking recipes. For example, you can toss fresh cilantro into tacos, sprinkle rosemary on roasted potatoes, or stir dill into yogurt for a refreshing dip. Herbal teas are another excellent way to enjoy the benefits of herbs; try steeping chamomile for relaxation or peppermint for digestion. You can also blend herbs into smoothies or use them to make infused oils and vinegars. For beginners, focus on one or two herbs to experiment with in your cooking, then gradually expand your repertoire. By consistently adding small amounts of herbs to your meals, you'll enhance both flavor and nutrition.

## HERBAL SUPPLEMENTS AND POWDERS

Herbal supplements and powders provide a convenient way to consume concentrated forms of herbs, but it's essential to approach them with caution. The U.S. Food and Drug Administration (FDA) does not regulate supplements as strictly as medications, which means their quality and efficacy can vary. To ensure you're getting a safe and effective product, look for third-party certifications such as USP, NSF, or ConsumerLab, which verify purity and potency. Research the brand's reputation, and prioritize products made from organic or sustainably sourced ingredients.

When purchasing herbal powders, such as turmeric or maca, check for freshness and avoid products with unnecessary fillers or additives. Trusted retailers, including reputable health food stores and established online vendors, are your best bet for high-quality products. Consult with a healthcare professional, especially if you're pregnant, nursing, or taking medications, to ensure the supplements are appropriate for you. By choosing supplements wisely and using them as part of a balanced diet, you can safely harness the benefits of herbal nutrition.

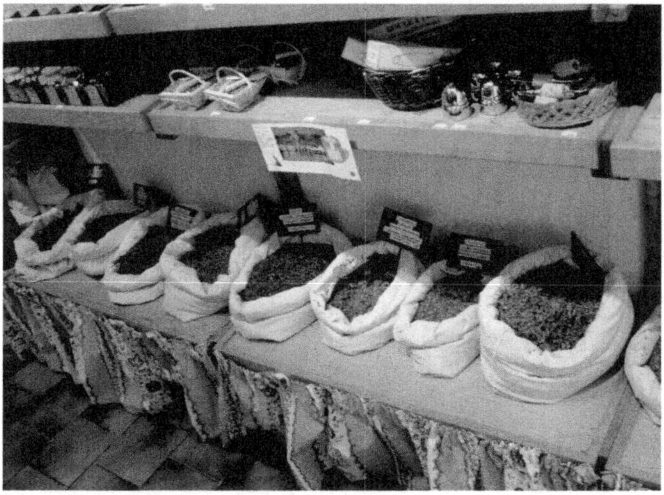

*Dried herbs*

# CHAPTER 8
# HERBAL REMEDIES FOR MENSTRUAL HEALTH

Supporting menstrual health is an essential aspect of holistic wellness. Herbs have been used for centuries to alleviate discomfort, regulate cycles, and promote hormonal balance. This chapter focuses on herbal remedies and lifestyle practices to support menstruation, including recipes for teas, tinctures, and soothing balms. By integrating these natural remedies, you can manage common menstrual concerns with ease and comfort.

**Understanding Menstrual Health**

Menstrual health involves the balance of hormones, proper blood circulation, and a well-functioning reproductive system. Discomfort during menstruation, such as cramps, bloating, and fatigue, often stems from inflammation or hormonal imbalances. Stress, diet, and lifestyle factors can also exacerbate symptoms. Incorporating herbs into your routine can help reduce pain, improve mood, and promote overall well-being during your cycle.

## HERBS FOR MENSTRUAL HEALTH

**Red Raspberry Leaf**

- **Benefits:** Supports uterine health, reduces cramps, and regulates menstrual flow.
- **Usage:** Brew as tea or combine with other herbs in infusions.

**Chasteberry**

- **Benefits:** Balances hormones and reduces symptoms of PMS, including mood swings and breast tenderness.
- **Usage:** Take as a tincture or in capsules.

**Ginger**

- **Benefits:** Anti-inflammatory properties help reduce cramps and bloating.
- **Usage:** Add to teas, soups, or smoothies.

**Cinnamon**

- **Benefits:** Improves blood circulation and reduces menstrual pain.
- **Usage:** Sprinkle on oatmeal or brew into a warm tea.

**Dong Quai**

- **Benefits:** Promotes blood flow and balances hormones.
- **Usage:** Take as a tea or tincture.

**Evening Primrose**

- **Benefits:** Alleviates cramps and supports hormonal balance.
- **Usage:** Use as an oil supplement or in topical applications.

**Peppermint**

- **Benefits:** Soothes nausea and reduces cramps.
- **Usage:** Brew as tea or add fresh leaves to water.

**Yarrow**

- **Benefits:** Reduces heavy bleeding and inflammation.
- **Usage:** Brew as tea or use in poultices.

## HERBAL TEAS FOR MENSTRUAL SUPPORT

### Soothing Raspberry Leaf Tea

*Ingredients*

- 1 tablespoon dried red raspberry leaves
- 1 teaspoon dried chamomile
- 1 teaspoon dried peppermint
- 1 cup boiling water

*Instructions*

Combine all herbs in a tea strainer.

Pour boiling water over the herbs and steep for 10 minutes.

Strain and sip warm.

*Where to Find Ingredients:* Red raspberry leaves, chamomile, and peppermint are available at herbal shops or online.

### Ginger and Cinnamon Comfort Tea

*Ingredients*

- 1-inch piece fresh ginger, sliced

- 1 cinnamon stick
- 1 teaspoon raw honey (optional)
- 1 cup boiling water

*Instructions*

Add ginger and cinnamon to boiling water.

Steep for 10 minutes, then strain.

Sweeten with honey if desired.

*Where to Find Ingredients:* Fresh ginger and cinnamon sticks can be found in grocery stores or spice shops.

**Hormone-Balancing Chasteberry Tea**

*Ingredients*

- 1 teaspoon dried chasteberry
- 1 teaspoon dried yarrow
- 1 cup boiling water

*Instructions*

Steep chasteberry and yarrow in boiling water for 10 minutes.

Strain and enjoy warm.

*Where to Find Ingredients:* Chasteberry and yarrow are available at herbal suppliers or online.

**Evening Primrose and Lemon Balm Tea**

*Ingredients*

- 1 teaspoon dried evening primrose flowers
- 1 teaspoon dried lemon balm
- 1 cup boiling water

*Instructions*

Combine herbs in a tea strainer and steep in boiling water for 10 minutes.

Strain and drink to reduce cramps and promote relaxation.

*Where to Find Ingredients:* Evening primrose and lemon balm can be found at health food stores or online.

**Dong Quai and Ginger Detox Tea**

*Ingredients*

- 1 teaspoon dried dong quai root
- 1-inch piece fresh ginger, sliced
- 1 cup boiling water

*Instructions*

Steep dong quai and ginger in boiling water for 10-15 minutes.

Strain and sip warm.

*Where to Find Ingredients:* Dong quai root and fresh ginger are available in herbal shops or grocery stores.

## TINCTURES AND BALMS FOR MENSTRUAL RELIEF

**Cramp-Relief Tincture**

*Ingredients*

- 1 cup dried red raspberry leaves
- 1 cup dried cramp bark
- 2 cups high-proof alcohol (such as vodka)

*Instructions*

Combine herbs in a sterilized glass jar.

Cover with alcohol and seal tightly.

Store in a dark, cool place for 4-6 weeks, shaking occasionally.

Strain and store in a dropper bottle. Take 1 teaspoon diluted in water during cramps.

*Where to Find Ingredients:* Red raspberry leaves and cramp bark can be purchased online or at herbal suppliers.

**Soothing Lavender and Peppermint Balm**

*Ingredients*

- 1/4 cup coconut oil
- 1 tablespoon beeswax
- 10 drops lavender essential oil
- 5 drops peppermint essential oil

*Instructions*

Melt coconut oil and beeswax in a double boiler.

Remove from heat and stir in essential oils.

Pour into a sterilized jar and let cool.

Apply to the lower abdomen to soothe cramps.

*Where to Find Ingredients:* Coconut oil and essential oils are available at health food stores or online.

## LIFESTYLE TIPS FOR MENSTRUAL HEALTH

- **Stay Hydrated:** Proper hydration reduces bloating and supports circulation.
- **Exercise Regularly:** Gentle activities like yoga or walking can relieve cramps and improve mood.

- **Eat Nutrient-Rich Foods:** Focus on magnesium-rich foods like leafy greens, nuts, and seeds to ease symptoms.
- **Practice Relaxation Techniques:** Deep breathing and meditation can help manage stress and reduce discomfort.

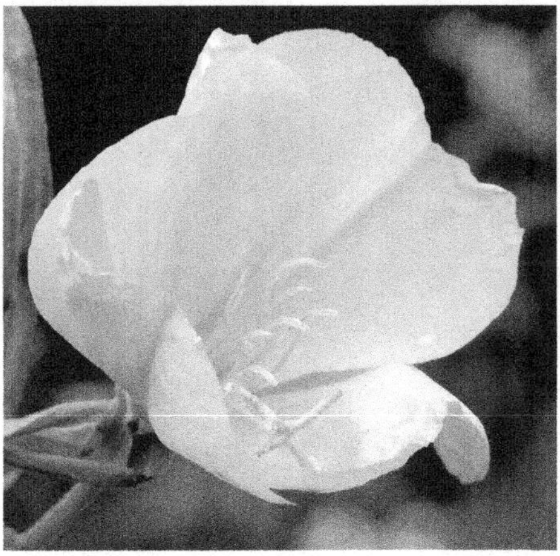

*Evening Primrose*

# CHAPTER 9
# HERBAL REMEDIES FOR GOUT

Gout is a form of arthritis caused by the buildup of uric acid crystals in the joints, leading to intense pain, inflammation, and swelling. It often affects the big toe but can occur in other joints as well. Lifestyle changes and herbal remedies can help manage gout by reducing inflammation, improving circulation, and lowering uric acid levels. This chapter explores effective herbal solutions, teas, tinctures, and lifestyle tips to ease gout symptoms and prevent future flare-ups.

**Understanding Gout**

Gout develops when the body produces too much uric acid or fails to eliminate it efficiently, resulting in crystal deposits in the joints. Common triggers include a diet high in purines (found in red meat, seafood, and alcohol), dehydration, and metabolic issues. Herbal remedies can provide natural relief by promoting uric acid excretion, reducing inflammation, and improving kidney function.

## HERBS FOR GOUT RELIEF

**Cherries**

- **Benefits:** Rich in antioxidants and anthocyanins that reduce uric acid and inflammation.
- **Usage:** Consume fresh or dried cherries daily or drink tart cherry juice.

**Dandelion**

- **Benefits:** Supports liver and kidney function, aiding in uric acid elimination.
- **Usage:** Brew as tea or use fresh leaves in salads.

**Celery Seed**

- **Benefits:** Promotes uric acid excretion and reduces joint inflammation.
- **Usage:** Take as a supplement or brew into tea.

**Nettle**

- **Benefits:** Anti-inflammatory properties help alleviate joint pain and swelling.
- **Usage:** Brew as tea or use dried nettle in soups.

**Turmeric**

- **Benefits:** Reduces inflammation and joint pain with its active compound, curcumin.
- **Usage:** Add to foods, teas, or take as a supplement.

**Ginger**

- **Benefits:** Improves circulation and reduces inflammation.
- **Usage:** Brew as tea or use fresh in cooking.

**Devil's Claw**

- **Benefits:** Alleviates joint pain and inflammation.
- **Usage:** Take as a tincture or in capsules.

**Milk Thistle**

- **Benefits:** Supports liver detoxification and uric acid metabolism.
- **Usage:** Brew as tea or take in capsule form.

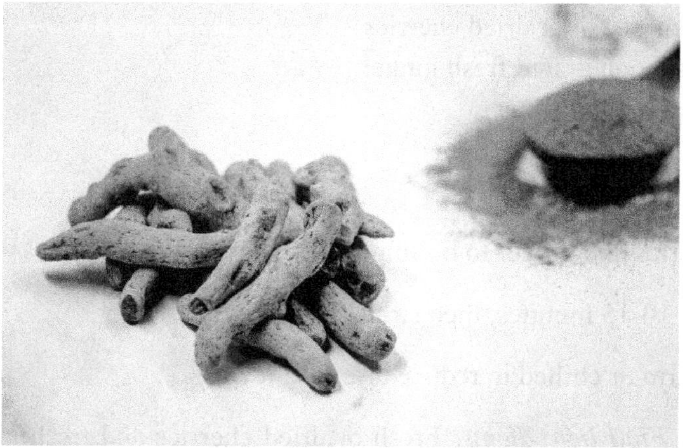

*Turmeric*

## HERBAL TEAS FOR GOUT RELIEF

**Dandelion and Nettle Detox Tea**

*Ingredients*

- 1 tablespoon dried dandelion root
- 1 tablespoon dried nettle leaves
- 1 cup boiling water

*Instructions*

Combine dandelion root and nettle leaves in a tea strainer.

Pour boiling water over the herbs and steep for 10 minutes.

Strain and sip warm to support kidney function and reduce inflammation.

*Where to Find Ingredients:* Dandelion root and nettle leaves are available at herbal shops or online.

**Cherry and Ginger Anti-Inflammatory Tea**

*Ingredients*

- 1/2 cup fresh or dried cherries
- 1 teaspoon grated fresh ginger
- 1 cup boiling water

*Instructions*

Add cherries and ginger to boiling water.

Steep for 10-15 minutes, then strain.

Drink warm or chilled to reduce uric acid levels.

*Where to Find Ingredients:* Fresh or dried cherries and fresh ginger can be found in grocery stores.

**Celery Seed and Lemon Tea**

*Ingredients*

- 1 teaspoon celery seeds
- Juice of 1/2 fresh lemon
- 1 cup boiling water

*Instructions*

Steep celery seeds in boiling water for 10 minutes.

Strain and stir in lemon juice.

Drink warm to promote uric acid excretion.

*Where to Find Ingredients:* Celery seeds and lemons are widely available in grocery stores.

**Turmeric and Cinnamon Joint Relief Tea**

*Ingredients*

- 1 teaspoon ground turmeric
- 1/2 teaspoon ground cinnamon
- 1 cup boiling water
- Honey (optional)

*Instructions*

Combine turmeric and cinnamon in a cup.

Pour boiling water over the mixture and steep for 10 minutes.

Strain and sweeten with honey if desired.

*Where to Find Ingredients:* Turmeric and cinnamon are available in the spice aisle of grocery stores.

**Milk Thistle and Peppermint Tea**

*Ingredients*

- 1 teaspoon dried milk thistle seeds
- 1 teaspoon dried peppermint leaves
- 1 cup boiling water

*Instructions*

Combine milk thistle seeds and peppermint in a tea strainer.

Steep in boiling water for 10 minutes.

Strain and sip warm to support detoxification.

*Where to Find Ingredients:* Milk thistle seeds and peppermint leaves can be purchased online or from herbal suppliers.

## TINCTURES AND TOPICAL REMEDIES FOR GOUT

**Celery Seed Tincture**

*Ingredients*

- 1 cup celery seeds
- 2 cups high-proof alcohol (such as vodka)

*Instructions*

Place celery seeds in a sterilized glass jar.

Cover with alcohol and seal tightly.

Store in a dark, cool place for 4-6 weeks, shaking occasionally.

Strain and store in a dropper bottle. Take 1 teaspoon diluted in water daily.

*Where to Find Ingredients:* Celery seeds can be found in the spice aisle or online.

**Cayenne Pain-Relief Balm**

*Ingredients*

- 1/4 cup coconut oil
- 1 tablespoon beeswax
- 1 teaspoon cayenne pepper powder

- 5 drops lavender essential oil

*Instructions*

Melt coconut oil and beeswax in a double boiler.

Stir in cayenne powder and lavender oil.

Pour into a sterilized jar and let cool.

Apply to affected joints as needed.

*Where to Find Ingredients:* Cayenne powder, coconut oil, and beeswax are available at health food stores or online.

## LIFESTYLE TIPS FOR MANAGING GOUT

- **Stay Hydrated:** Drinking plenty of water helps flush uric acid from the body.
- **Limit Purine-Rich Foods:** Reduce intake of red meat, seafood, and alcohol.
- **Maintain a Healthy Weight:** Excess weight can increase uric acid levels.
- **Exercise Regularly:** Gentle activities like swimming or walking support joint health.
- **Avoid Sugary Drinks:** High-fructose beverages can exacerbate gout symptoms.

# CHAPTER 10
# HAIR CARE

## HERBS FOR HAIR HEALTH: IN-DEPTH PROFILES

Our hair requires proper nourishment, circulation, and care, and herbs provide an excellent and natural means to address all these needs. Here, we'll go deeper into the individual herbs, exploring their active compounds, unique properties, and benefits for different hair conditions.

**Rosemary**

*Overview*

Rosemary is a perennial herb native to the Mediterranean and is widely used in both culinary and medicinal applications. Its rich aroma and active compounds, such as rosmarinic acid and ursolic acid, make it a powerful ally for hair health.

*Key Benefits for Hair*

- **Stimulates Hair Growth:** Rosemary has been shown to promote hair growth by stimulating blood circulation to the scalp. This improved circulation brings more nutrients to the hair follicles, supporting healthy growth.

- **Fights Dandruff:** It helps reduce dandruff and flakiness by promoting the renewal of skin cells on the scalp.
- **Strengthens Hair:** Rosemary contains antioxidants that help protect hair from environmental stressors, strengthening the strands and preventing damage.

*How It Works*

Rosemary enhances blood circulation in the scalp, nourishing the follicles. It is particularly useful for combating hair thinning, dandruff, and scalp irritation. Rosemary's antiseptic properties help prevent scalp infections and can help control oily scalp conditions by balancing oil production.

*Where to Find Rosemary*

Rosemary is easy to find at health food stores, herb shops, or even in your own garden. You can purchase dried rosemary, rosemary essential oil, or live plants to grow at home. For fresh rosemary, you can typically find it at grocery stores in the herb section.

**Nettle**

*Overview*

Nettle is a robust herb often found in temperate regions around the world. Its leaves contain a wealth of vitamins and minerals, including vitamins A, C, K, iron, and silica, all of which are important for maintaining healthy hair.

*Key Benefits for Hair*

- **Promotes Hair Growth:** Nettle is believed to stimulate hair follicles, encouraging new hair growth. Its high iron content helps prevent hair loss due to iron deficiency.

- **Improves Hair Texture:** Nettle's silica content strengthens hair strands, making them more resilient to breakage.
- **Balances the Scalp:** Nettle helps balance the scalp's natural oils, reducing excessive dryness or oiliness.

*How It Works*

Nettle's anti-inflammatory properties reduce scalp irritation and can relieve itchy, flaky skin. The presence of iron and silica strengthens the hair and prevents it from thinning. This herb also promotes overall scalp health, preventing dandruff and other scalp conditions.

*Where to Find Nettle*

Nettle can be found in many health food stores, particularly in dried or powdered form. It's often sold in capsules or as a tea blend. You can also forage for it in the wild, but make sure to handle it carefully as its leaves are covered in stinging hairs. Nettle is also available online from reputable herbal shops.

**Horsetail**

*Overview*

Horsetail is an ancient plant that grows in moist, temperate regions around the world. It's known for its high silica content, which is crucial for maintaining the structural integrity of hair, skin, and nails.

*Key Benefits for Hair*

- **Strengthens Hair Strands:** The high silica content in horsetail helps to strengthen hair by improving the formation of collagen, a protein that supports hair structure.
- **Prevents Breakage:** Horsetail is commonly used to prevent hair breakage by improving the elasticity and strength of hair.
- **Stimulates Growth:** Horsetail helps promote circulation to the scalp and, over time, can stimulate hair follicles, encouraging growth.

*How It Works*

Silica is vital for building strong hair strands and maintaining their smoothness. Horsetail's silica content not only strengthens hair but also prevents premature hair loss and supports overall scalp health. It's often used for its ability to reduce hair thinning and rejuvenate fragile strands.

*Where to Find Horsetail*

Horsetail can be purchased in dried form at health food stores or herbal shops. It is often found as a loose leaf or in capsule form. Horsetail is also available in some online herbal shops. If you're interested in growing your own, horsetail can be cultivated in a wet, shaded area in your garden.

**Lavender**

*Overview*

Lavender is one of the most well-known herbs in the world, not only for its calming scent but also for its extensive medicinal properties. Lavender essential oil is widely used in aromatherapy and beauty products.

*Key Benefits for Hair*

- **Stimulates Follicles for Growth:** Lavender has been shown to help increase hair growth by stimulating hair follicles. It is especially useful in preventing hair loss related to stress.
- **Balances Scalp Health:** Lavender has antifungal and antibacterial properties, which make it ideal for treating scalp infections and imbalances.
- **Soothes Scalp Irritation:** Lavender helps calm irritation and inflammation in the scalp, reducing conditions like dandruff and itching.

*How It Works*

Lavender improves blood flow to the scalp, promoting healthy hair growth. Its calming properties reduce stress, which is one of the common causes of hair loss. Lavender oil also helps regulate the production of sebum (the scalp's natural oil), preventing both oily scalp and dry flakes.

*Where to Find Lavender*

Lavender essential oil is available in most health food stores and online. You can also find dried lavender flowers in herbal shops, where it is often sold as part of a tea blend or as an ingredient in beauty products. Growing lavender in your garden is a great option if you want to have a fresh supply on hand.

**Peppermint**

*Overview*

Peppermint is a hybrid plant created by crossing watermint and spearmint. It's well-known for its cooling and refreshing qualities, and it is packed with menthol, which has a wide range of beneficial properties for hair health.

*Key Benefits for Hair*

- **Promotes Circulation:** The menthol in peppermint helps increase circulation to the scalp, stimulating hair follicles and encouraging growth.
- **Reduces Itchiness:** Peppermint's cooling effect helps alleviate itching and irritation on the scalp, which can be caused by dryness or dandruff.
- **Clears Oily Build-up:** Peppermint helps balance scalp oil production and clears excess oils and buildup that can contribute to clogged follicles and hair thinning.

*How It Works*

Peppermint stimulates the blood vessels beneath the scalp, increasing nutrient delivery to hair follicles, which helps promote healthy growth. It also has astringent properties that help reduce oil production, making it an excellent choice for those with oily hair or scalp.

*Where to Find Peppermint*

Peppermint essential oil can be found at health food stores or online. You can also purchase dried peppermint leaves, which are often sold in bulk at herb shops. Growing peppermint is easy, as it thrives in a variety of climates and can be propagated from cuttings or seeds.

## DIY HAIR TREATMENTS: RECIPES FOR HEALTHY HAIR

Let's now dive into some practical, easy-to-make hair care recipes using the herbs mentioned above.

### Rosemary & Nettle Hair Growth Rinse

This invigorating hair rinse helps stimulate hair growth while also balancing scalp health. The combination of rosemary and nettle is particularly effective for encouraging hair to grow strong and thick.

*Ingredients*

- 2 tablespoons dried rosemary
- 2 tablespoons dried nettle leaves
- 2 cups water

*Instructions*

Boil the water and pour it over the dried rosemary and nettle leaves in a heatproof container.

Cover the container and let the herbs steep for 15-20 minutes.

Strain the liquid to remove the herbs.

Once cooled to room temperature, use the rinse after shampooing your hair. Pour the rinse over your scalp and hair, making sure to thoroughly soak the roots and tips.

Gently massage your scalp and let the rinse sit for 5-10 minutes before rinsing with cool water.

*Where to Find Ingredients:* Rosemary and nettle can be purchased at health food stores, herb shops, or online. Nettle is often available as a loose leaf or in capsules, and rosemary is widely available in dried or essential oil form.

**Lavender & Horsetail Scalp Soothing Oil**

This soothing oil helps calm an irritated scalp, stimulate hair growth, and prevent hair breakage. Horsetail's silica strengthens hair, while lavender's anti-inflammatory properties help soothe the scalp.

*Ingredients*

- 3 tablespoons dried horsetail
- 2 tablespoons dried lavender flowers
- 1/4 cup jojoba oil (or coconut oil)

*Instructions*

Combine the dried horsetail and lavender flowers in a small glass jar or bottle.

Pour the jojoba oil over the herbs, ensuring that the herbs are completely submerged.

Seal the jar and let it sit in a cool, dark place for 1-2 weeks, shaking gently every couple of days to mix.

After the steeping period, strain the herbs from the oil and store the infused oil in a clean bottle.

Massage the oil into your scalp before bedtime. Leave it on overnight, and wash your hair with a gentle shampoo the next morning.

*Where to Find Ingredients:* Lavender and horsetail are available at most health food stores, online herb shops, and some specialty stores. You can also grow your own lavender and purchase horsetail in dried or capsule form.

**Peppermint Scalp Cooling Treatment**

This peppermint treatment helps reduce oiliness and irritation on the scalp, leaving it feeling fresh and revitalized.

*Ingredients*

- 6-8 drops peppermint essential oil
- 2 tablespoons carrier oil (coconut oil, jojoba oil, or argan oil)
- 1 tablespoon honey (optional for added moisture)

*Instructions*

Mix the peppermint essential oil with the carrier oil of your choice.

If using, add the honey and stir until combined.

Massage the oil into your scalp for 5-10 minutes, focusing on areas that feel itchy or oily.

Leave the treatment on for 30-45 minutes and then wash out with a gentle shampoo.

*Where to Find Ingredients:* Peppermint essential oil is widely available at health food stores, online marketplaces, or specialty stores. Carrier oils such as coconut or jojoba are commonly found in grocery stores or beauty stores. Honey can be sourced from local farmers' markets or grocery stores.

**Conclusion**

In this chapter, we've explored the remarkable power of herbs for hair care. By incorporating herbs like rosemary, nettle, horsetail, lavender, and peppermint into your hair care routine, you can enhance your hair's strength, growth, and overall health. The recipes provided are easy to make, and many of the herbs can be found at your local health food store, herbalist, or online.

By using these herbal remedies regularly, you can nurture your hair from the roots to the tips, naturally supporting its growth, texture, and shine without the harsh chemicals often found in commercial products.

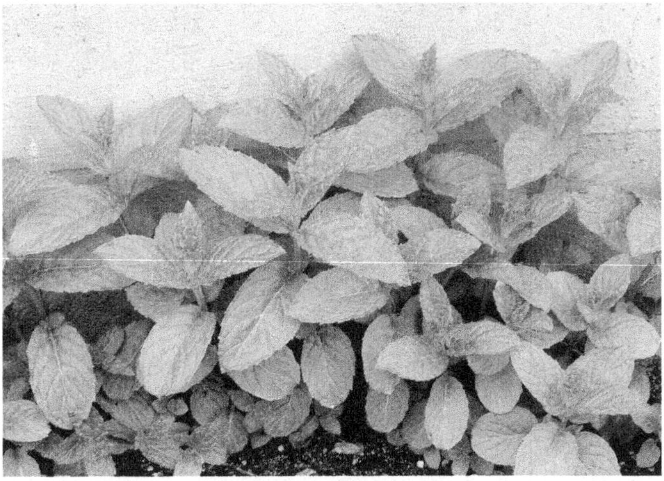

*Peppermint*

# CHAPTER II
# FACE CARE

## HERBS FOR FACIAL HEALTH

Caring for the skin on our face requires delicate balance. The skin here is often more sensitive and susceptible to environmental damage, aging, and common concerns like acne, dryness, or oiliness. Herbal remedies for face care are an excellent way to nourish, treat, and protect the skin naturally. In this chapter, we explore the best herbs for maintaining clear, healthy, and youthful skin, followed by a variety of recipes for masks, scrubs, toners, and anti-aging treatments.

**Aloe Vera**

*Overview:* Aloe vera is one of the most well-known herbs in skincare. This succulent plant is renowned for its soothing and moisturizing properties, which make it a go-to for treating sunburn, dry skin, and inflammation. Aloe vera contains vitamins A, C, and E, along with antioxidants and enzymes that help rejuvenate the skin.

*Key Benefits for the Face*

- **Soothes Inflammation:** Aloe vera is excellent for calming inflamed or irritated skin, making it ideal for acne-prone skin or sensitive skin.
- **Hydrates Skin:** It deeply hydrates the skin without making it greasy, making it great for all skin types.
- **Promotes Healing:** Aloe vera accelerates the healing process of skin wounds, cuts, and burns.

*Where to Find Aloe Vera:* Fresh aloe vera leaves can often be found in health food stores or farmers' markets. You can also purchase aloe vera gel or juice at most natural grocery stores or online. For topical applications, fresh aloe vera is preferable, but commercial gels work well if they are free of additives.

**Chamomile**

*Overview:* Chamomile is a flowering herb known for its calming and anti-inflammatory properties. The gentle nature of chamomile makes it an excellent choice for sensitive skin, including for those suffering from conditions like rosacea or eczema.

*Key Benefits for the Face*

- **Soothes Irritation:** Chamomile's anti-inflammatory properties make it excellent for calming redness, irritation, and puffiness on the skin.
- **Gentle on Sensitive Skin:** It is non-irritating, making it perfect for those with delicate or reactive skin.
- **Reduces Under-Eye Puffiness:** Chamomile's ability to reduce swelling and promote circulation makes it an effective ingredient for reducing puffiness, especially around the eyes.

*Where to Find Chamomile:* Chamomile is commonly available as dried flowers in health food stores, herbal shops, or online. You can also purchase chamomile essential oil, which is often found in the skincare section of natural product stores.

**Lavender**

*Overview:* Lavender is not just a soothing herb for the senses but also a powerful remedy for skin health. Known for its antibacterial, antifungal, and anti-inflammatory properties, lavender is a great herb to use in facial care, especially for acne and oily skin.

*Key Benefits for the Face*

- **Treats Acne:** Lavender's antimicrobial properties help combat acne-causing bacteria, making it an effective choice for acne-prone skin.
- **Calms Redness:** Lavender has anti-inflammatory effects, which can reduce redness and swelling on the skin.
- **Anti-aging:** Lavender has antioxidants that help protect the skin from free radical damage, which contributes to aging.

*Where to Find Lavender:* Lavender is widely available in health food stores, herb shops, or online. You can use either dried lavender flowers or lavender essential oil. For topical use, ensure the essential oil is diluted with a carrier oil to avoid skin irritation.

**Rose**

*Overview:* Rose is known for its luxurious fragrance, but it also boasts impressive skincare benefits. Rose contains high levels of vitamin C and antioxidants, which help protect the skin from damage and support healthy aging.

*Key Benefits for the Face*

- **Hydrates Skin:** Rose helps replenish moisture in the skin, making it an excellent ingredient for dry or mature skin.
- **Anti-aging:** The antioxidants in rose petals help fight free radical damage, which accelerates the aging process.

- **Reduces Redness:** Rose can help calm inflamed and irritated skin, reducing redness and promoting a more even complexion.

*Where to Find Rose:* Fresh rose petals can be purchased from farmers' markets or grown at home. Rose essential oil and rose water are available at many health food stores or online. Be sure to choose high-quality, organic rose water for the best results in skincare.

**Witch Hazel**

*Overview:* Witch hazel is a natural astringent and one of the best toning herbs for the skin. It helps tighten the skin, reduce inflammation, and minimize pores, making it an essential ingredient for those with oily or acne-prone skin.

*Key Benefits for the Face*

- **Reduces Acne:** Witch hazel's astringent properties make it effective in reducing acne breakouts by removing excess oil and preventing clogged pores.
- **Tightens Pores:** It helps minimize the appearance of pores by tightening the skin and promoting a smoother complexion.
- **Calms Skin Irritation:** Witch hazel can also reduce redness and swelling from skin irritations, making it useful for sensitive or inflamed skin.

*Where to Find Witch Hazel:* Witch hazel extract is readily available in most pharmacies, health food stores, and online. When choosing witch hazel, look for a product with minimal alcohol content to avoid drying out the skin.

## HERBAL FACE MASKS: RECIPES FOR GLOWING SKIN

Herbal face masks can help nourish the skin with natural ingredients. Below are recipes that utilize the herbs we've just explored, targeting different skin needs.

**Aloe Vera & Honey Hydrating Mask**

This mask is perfect for dry skin, offering hydration and soothing relief.

*Ingredients*

- 2 tablespoons aloe vera gel (fresh or store-bought)
- 1 tablespoon raw honey

*Instructions*

Mix the aloe vera gel and honey in a bowl until smooth.

Apply the mixture to your face, avoiding the eyes.

Leave the mask on for 15-20 minutes.

Rinse off with lukewarm water.

*Where to Find Ingredients:* You can find aloe vera gel in most health food stores, and raw honey can be sourced from local farms or health markets.

**Chamomile & Oatmeal Calming Mask**

Chamomile's soothing properties, combined with the gentle exfoliation of oatmeal, make this mask perfect for sensitive skin.

*Ingredients*

- 2 tablespoons chamomile tea (cooled)
- 1 tablespoon oatmeal (ground)
- 1 teaspoon honey

*Instructions*

Brew chamomile tea and let it cool.

In a bowl, combine the cooled tea, oatmeal, and honey.

Stir until you form a paste.

Apply the paste to your face, leave on for 15 minutes, and rinse off with warm water.

*Where to Find Ingredients:* Chamomile tea is available in most grocery stores, and oatmeal can be found in any supermarket. Raw honey can be purchased at health food stores.

**Lavender & Clay Detoxifying Mask**

Lavender's antibacterial properties combined with the deep-cleansing action of clay make this mask a great choice for acne-prone skin.

*Ingredients*

- 1 tablespoon clay powder (bentonite or kaolin)
- 4 drops lavender essential oil
- Water to form a paste

*Instructions*

Mix the clay powder with enough water to form a thick paste.

Add lavender essential oil to the paste and stir.

Apply to your face, leaving it on for 10-15 minutes.

Rinse with warm water.

*Where to Find Ingredients:* Clay powder and lavender essential oil are both available at health food stores, online herbal shops, and beauty supply stores.

**Rose & Yogurt Brightening Mask**

This mask helps brighten the skin and reduce redness with the calming properties of rose and the skin-brightening benefits of yogurt.

*Ingredients:=*

- 1 tablespoon rose water
- 2 tablespoons plain yogurt

- 1 teaspoon honey

*Instructions*

Mix the rose water, yogurt, and honey in a bowl.

Apply the mixture to your face and leave on for 15-20 minutes.

Rinse off with lukewarm water.

*Where to Find Ingredients:* Rose water is available at most health food stores, and plain yogurt can be purchased at any grocery store.

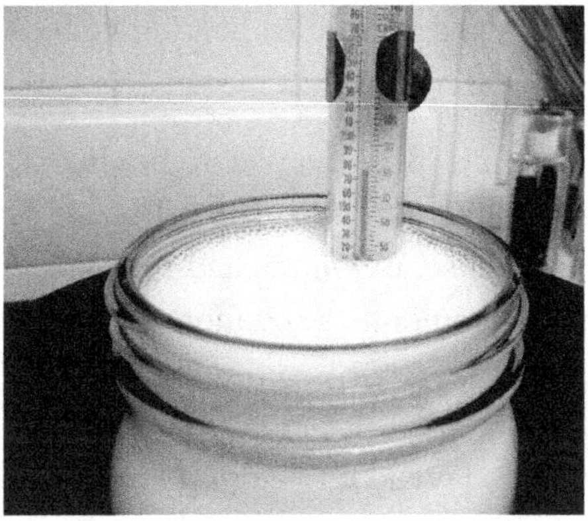

*Yogurt*

**Witch Hazel & Green Tea Clarifying Mask**

Witch hazel helps tighten pores, while green tea offers antioxidant protection for clearer, smoother skin.

*Ingredients*

- 1 tablespoon witch hazel extract
- 1 tablespoon brewed green tea (cooled)
- 1 tablespoon honey

*Instructions*

Mix all the ingredients in a small bowl until smooth.

Apply the mask to your face and leave it on for 15 minutes.

Rinse off with warm water.

*Where to Find Ingredients:* Witch hazel is available in pharmacies and health food stores, and green tea can be found in any grocery store.

## HERBAL SCRUBS FOR THE FACE: RECIPES FOR RADIANT SKIN

Facial scrubs exfoliate dead skin cells, helping your skin to look brighter and smoother.

Exfoliating your face is a key step in removing dead skin cells and allowing fresh skin to shine through. The following herbal scrub recipes are designed to help cleanse, exfoliate, and rejuvenate the skin naturally, making your complexion smoother and more vibrant.

**Lavender & Brown Sugar Exfoliating Scrub**

This soothing scrub uses lavender to calm the skin while the brown sugar gently exfoliates, making it perfect for sensitive skin types.

*Ingredients*

- 2 tablespoons brown sugar
- 1 tablespoon lavender essential oil
- 1 tablespoon olive oil

*Instructions*

Combine the brown sugar, lavender essential oil, and olive oil in a small bowl.

Mix well until the sugar is evenly coated.

Gently massage the scrub onto your damp face in circular motions for 2-3 minutes.

Rinse with warm water and pat your face dry.

*Where to Find Ingredients:* Brown sugar, olive oil, and lavender essential oil are readily available in grocery stores, health food shops, and online.

**Oatmeal & Chamomile Soothing Scrub**

Oatmeal is a gentle exfoliant, and chamomile helps to soothe and calm irritated skin. This scrub is perfect for those with sensitive or red skin.

*Ingredients*

- 2 tablespoons ground oatmeal
- 1 tablespoon dried chamomile flowers
- 1 tablespoon honey
- 1-2 tablespoons warm water

*Instructions*

Grind the chamomile flowers into a fine powder using a coffee grinder or mortar and pestle.

Mix the ground oatmeal, chamomile powder, and honey in a bowl.

Add warm water slowly to create a paste.

Gently massage the paste onto your face in circular motions for 2-3 minutes.

Rinse with lukewarm water.

*Where to Find Ingredients:* You can find dried chamomile flowers and oatmeal at any health food store, herbalist, or online. Honey is typically available at grocery stores and farmer's markets.

**Rose & Almond Scrub for Soft Skin**

Almonds provide a rich source of Vitamin E and fatty acids, perfect for moisturizing the skin. Combined with the soothing properties of rose petals, this scrub leaves your skin feeling soft and nourished.

*Ingredients*

- 2 tablespoons ground almonds
- 1 tablespoon dried rose petals (crushed)
- 1 teaspoon honey
- 1 tablespoon coconut oil

*Instructions*

Crush the dried rose petals and mix them with ground almonds.

Add honey and coconut oil to the mixture and stir until it forms a thick paste.

Gently massage the scrub into your face for 2-3 minutes, focusing on areas of dryness.

Rinse off with warm water.

*Where to Find Ingredients:* Ground almonds and dried rose petals can be purchased at health food stores, herbalists, or online. Coconut oil and honey are commonly found in most supermarkets.

**Coffee & Coconut Scrub for Brightness**

Coffee grounds are an excellent exfoliant that removes dead skin cells, while coconut oil hydrates and moisturizes, making this scrub ideal for dry and dull skin.

*Ingredients*

- 2 tablespoons coffee grounds (fresh or used)
- 1 tablespoon coconut oil
- 1 teaspoon honey

*Instructions*

Combine coffee grounds, coconut oil, and honey in a bowl.

Mix until the scrub has a smooth, thick consistency.

Gently massage onto damp skin, focusing on the areas that need exfoliation.

Rinse off with warm water.

*Where to Find Ingredients:* Coffee grounds, coconut oil, and honey are readily available in grocery stores or online. If you're using used coffee grounds, just ensure they are cool and free of liquid.

**Turmeric & Sugar Scrub for Glowing Skin**

Turmeric has brightening and anti-inflammatory properties, while sugar serves as a natural exfoliant. This scrub is especially useful for uneven skin tone and dullness.

*Ingredients*

- 2 tablespoons white sugar
- 1 teaspoon turmeric powder
- 1 tablespoon yogurt or honey

*Instructions*

Mix the sugar and turmeric in a small bowl.

Add yogurt or honey and stir until it forms a smooth paste.

Gently massage onto your face, especially focusing on areas with uneven skin tone.

Rinse off thoroughly with lukewarm water.

*Where to Find Ingredients:* Turmeric, white sugar, and honey can be found at most supermarkets. Yogurt is widely available at grocery stores.

**Green Tea & Honey Exfoliating Scrub**

Green tea's antioxidants help protect the skin, and combined with honey and sugar, it forms an excellent scrub to exfoliate and revitalize the face.

*Ingredients*

- 2 tablespoons sugar
- 1 tablespoon green tea (cooled)
- 1 tablespoon honey

*Instructions*

Brew green tea and allow it to cool.

Mix the sugar with honey and green tea to form a paste.

Massage the scrub onto your face for 2-3 minutes.

Rinse with cool water.

*Where to Find Ingredients:* Sugar, honey, and green tea are easily available in grocery stores, and you can find them in various organic forms in health food stores.

**Lavender & Sea Salt Scrub for Smooth Skin**

This scrub uses lavender for relaxation and sea salt for a deep exfoliation, helping you achieve smooth, glowing skin.

*Ingredients*

- 1 tablespoon sea salt
- 1 tablespoon lavender essential oil
- 1 tablespoon olive oil

*Instructions*

Mix the sea salt, lavender essential oil, and olive oil.

Gently apply the mixture to your face in small, circular motions for 2-3 minutes.

Rinse off with warm water.

*Where to Find Ingredients:* Sea salt, lavender essential oil, and olive oil are available at most supermarkets, health stores, or online.

**Papaya & Sugar Exfoliating Mask**

Papaya contains enzymes that naturally exfoliate the skin, while sugar provides physical exfoliation. Together, they help reveal a fresh complexion.

*Ingredients*

- 2 tablespoons fresh papaya (mashed)
- 1 tablespoon sugar

*Instructions*

Mash the papaya into a smooth paste.

Add the sugar and mix well.

Gently massage the mixture into your face for 2-3 minutes.

Rinse thoroughly with warm water.

*Where to Find Ingredients:* Fresh papayas can be found at most grocery stores, and sugar is available everywhere.

**Coconut & Mint Scrub for a Refreshing Cleanse**

Mint has cooling and antibacterial properties, while coconut oil moisturizes the skin. This scrub is refreshing and perfect for oily skin types.

*Ingredients:*

- 2 tablespoons shredded coconut
- 1 tablespoon fresh mint leaves (finely chopped)

- 1 tablespoon honey

*Instructions:*

Combine the shredded coconut, chopped mint leaves, and honey.

Mix thoroughly and gently scrub the mixture onto your damp skin.

Rinse off with lukewarm water.

*Where to Find Ingredients:* Coconut, honey, and mint leaves are easy to find in your local grocery store or farmer's market.

**Cinnamon & Honey Exfoliating Mask**

Cinnamon helps with circulation and promotes collagen production, while honey moisturizes and heals. This scrub is great for rejuvenating your skin.

*Ingredients*

- 1 tablespoon cinnamon powder
- 1 tablespoon honey

*Instructions*

Mix the cinnamon powder with honey until smooth.

Apply to your face, gently massaging in circular motions for a few minutes.

Leave on for 5 minutes, then rinse off with warm water.

*Where to Find Ingredients:* Cinnamon and honey are available in supermarkets, spice shops, and health food stores.

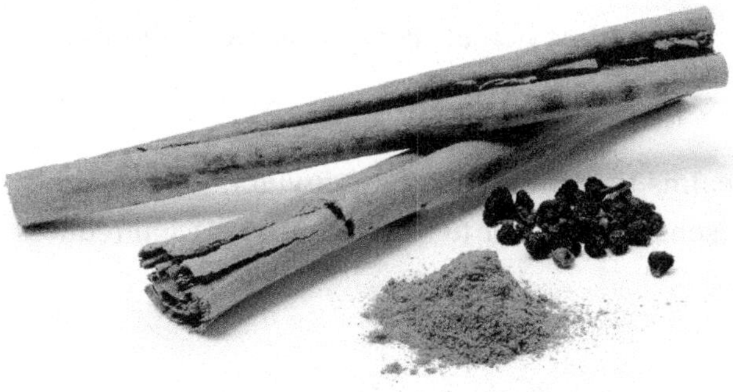

*Cinnamon*

## HERBAL STEAMS AND TONERS: RECIPES FOR CLEAR, BALANCED SKIN

Facial steams and toners are great for opening pores, clearing impurities, and providing deep hydration. Here are recipes to make your own custom steams and toners at home.

**Lavender & Rose Facial Steam**

Lavender's calming properties and rose's moisturizing abilities make this steam ideal for soothing and hydrating your skin.

*Ingredients*

- 1 tablespoon dried lavender flowers
- 1 tablespoon dried rose petals
- 4 cups boiling water

*Instructions*

Place the lavender and rose petals into a heatproof bowl.

Pour the boiling water over the herbs.

Lean over the bowl, covering your head with a towel to trap the steam. Steam your face for 10-15 minutes.

*Where to Find Ingredients:* Both lavender and rose petals can be found at health food stores, online herbal shops, or grown at home.

**Chamomile & Mint Facial Steam**

Chamomile calms the skin, while mint invigorates and cools. This steam is perfect for sensitive skin or to relieve puffiness and redness.

*Ingredients*

- 1 tablespoon dried chamomile flowers
- 1 tablespoon fresh mint leaves
- 4 cups boiling water

*Instructions*

Place chamomile flowers and mint leaves in a bowl.

Pour the boiling water over the herbs.

Lean over the bowl, covering your head with a towel to trap the steam. Steam for 10-15 minutes.

*Where to Find Ingredients:* Chamomile flowers and mint are available at health food stores, online herbal shops, and farmer's markets.

**Green Tea & Lemon Facial Steam**

Green tea's antioxidants help protect the skin, while lemon brightens and tightens. This steam helps refresh the skin and minimize pores.

*Ingredients*

- 1 green tea bag
- 1-2 lemon slices
- 4 cups boiling water

*Instructions*

Place the green tea bag and lemon slices in a bowl.

Pour boiling water over the ingredients.

Steam your face for 10-15 minutes.

*Where to Find Ingredients:* Green tea and lemons are easy to find in any supermarket or health food store.

**Rosemary & Eucalyptus Steam**

Rosemary helps increase circulation, while eucalyptus clears congestion and revitalizes the skin. This steam is perfect for tired, stressed skin.

*Ingredients:*

- 1 tablespoon dried rosemary
- 1-2 eucalyptus leaves
- 4 cups boiling water

*Instructions:*

Add the rosemary and eucalyptus to a heatproof bowl.

Pour the boiling water over the herbs.

Place your face over the steam and cover your head with a towel. Steam for 10-15 minutes.

*Where to Find Ingredients:* Rosemary and eucalyptus leaves are available at health food stores or online herbal shops.

## ANTI-AGING HERB RECIPES

As we age, the skin naturally loses collagen and elasticity, leading to fine lines and wrinkles. Fortunately, herbs can provide essential nutrients and antioxidants that fight these signs of aging.

**Calendula & Lavender Facial Steam**

Calendula is well-known for its healing properties, especially for inflamed or irritated skin, while lavender calms and promotes relaxation. This steam is ideal for soothing sensitive or inflamed skin.

*Ingredients*

- 1 tablespoon dried calendula flowers
- 1 tablespoon dried lavender flowers
- 4 cups boiling water

*Instructions*

Place the calendula and lavender flowers in a bowl.

Pour boiling water over the herbs.

Cover your head with a towel, trapping the steam, and lean over the bowl for 10-15 minutes.

*Where to Find Ingredients:* Calendula and lavender flowers can be found in health food stores, online herbal shops, or farmer's markets.

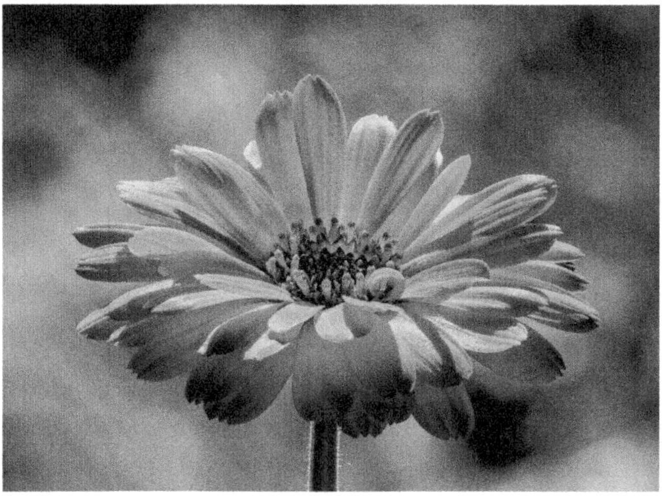

*Calendula*

**Hibiscus & Rose Facial Steam**

Hibiscus is rich in antioxidants, while rose water is known for its moisturizing and soothing properties. Together, they provide a rejuvenating steam that revitalizes the skin.

*Ingredients*

- 1 tablespoon dried hibiscus flowers
- 1 tablespoon rose water
- 4 cups boiling water

*Instructions*

Place the hibiscus flowers in a heatproof bowl.

Add rose water and pour in boiling water.

Steam your face for 10-15 minutes, keeping your head covered with a towel to trap the steam.

*Where to Find Ingredients:* Hibiscus flowers and rose water are available at most health food stores or online.

**Ginger & Lemon Steam for Radiance**

Ginger has natural antibacterial properties, and lemon is packed with Vitamin C, which brightens and tones the skin. This steam is perfect for dull or uneven skin tone.

*Ingredients*

- 1 tablespoon grated fresh ginger
- 1 lemon (sliced)
- 4 cups boiling water

*Instructions*

Grate fresh ginger and slice the lemon.

Add the ginger and lemon to a heatproof bowl and pour boiling water over them.

Steam your face for 10-15 minutes.

*Where to Find Ingredients:* Fresh ginger and lemons are available in grocery stores and health food stores.

**Sage & Rosemary Facial Steam**

Sage is a powerful herb known for its antibacterial properties, while rosemary helps improve circulation and promote healthy skin. This steam works wonders for those with acne-prone or oily skin.

*Ingredients*

- 1 tablespoon dried sage
- 1 tablespoon dried rosemary
- 4 cups boiling water

*Instructions*

Place the dried sage and rosemary in a bowl.

Pour boiling water over the herbs and cover your head with a towel.

Lean over the bowl for 10-15 minutes to let the steam open your pores.

*Where to Find Ingredients:* Sage and rosemary can be found at health food stores, herb shops, and online.

**Mint & Green Tea Facial Steam**

Green tea provides antioxidant protection, while mint adds a refreshing element that cools and tones the skin. This steam is perfect for relieving tired, puffy skin and reducing inflammation.

*Ingredients*

- 1 tablespoon dried mint leaves
- 1 green tea bag (or 1 tablespoon loose leaf)

- 4 cups boiling water

*Instructions*

Add the mint leaves and green tea to a bowl.

Pour boiling water over the herbs and cover your head with a towel to trap the steam.

Steam for 10-15 minutes.

*Where to Find Ingredients:* Mint and green tea are available at grocery stores, health food stores, and online.

**Jasmine & Ylang Ylang Steam for a Luxurious Treatment**

Jasmine is known for its ability to promote skin elasticity, while ylang ylang is great for balancing the skin's oil production. Together, these herbs offer a luxurious steam treatment that leaves skin feeling soft, moisturized, and fresh.

*Ingredients*

- 1 tablespoon dried jasmine flowers
- 1 tablespoon ylang ylang essential oil
- 4 cups boiling water

*Instructions*

Add dried jasmine flowers to a bowl.

Pour boiling water over the flowers, then add a few drops of ylang ylang essential oil.

Lean over the bowl, covered with a towel, for 10-15 minutes to let the steam open pores and nourish the skin.

*Where to Find Ingredients:* Jasmine flowers and ylang ylang essential oil are available at health food stores, herbal shops, and online.

**Elderflower & Lemon Balm Steam**

Elderflower is known for its calming and skin-soothing properties, while lemon balm helps to refresh and tone the skin. This steam is excellent for calming irritated skin and promoting relaxation.

*Ingredients*

- 1 tablespoon dried elderflower
- 1 tablespoon dried lemon balm
- 4 cups boiling water

*Instructions*

Add dried elderflower and lemon balm to a heatproof bowl.

Pour the boiling water over the herbs and cover your head with a towel.

Steam for 10-15 minutes.

*Where to Find Ingredients:* Elderflower and lemon balm can be found in health food stores, herbal suppliers, and online.

**Nettle & Rose Facial Steam for Sensitive Skin**

Nettle is rich in vitamins and minerals, while rose provides soothing and anti-inflammatory properties. This steam is perfect for anyone with sensitive or reactive skin.

*Ingredients*

- 1 tablespoon dried nettle leaves
- 1 tablespoon dried rose petals
- 4 cups boiling water

*Instructions*

Place the nettle leaves and rose petals in a bowl.

Pour boiling water over the herbs and cover with a towel to trap the steam.

Steam your face for 10-15 minutes.

*Where to Find Ingredients:* Nettle and rose petals can be sourced from health food stores, herb shops, or online.

**Lemon Verbena & Thyme Facial Steam**

Lemon verbena has an uplifting, citrus scent that helps with brightening, while thyme has antibacterial properties that can help reduce acne. This steam is great for dull, acne-prone skin.

*Ingredients*

- 1 tablespoon dried lemon verbena
- 1 tablespoon dried thyme
- 4 cups boiling water

*Instructions*

Add the lemon verbena and thyme to a heatproof bowl.

Pour boiling water over the herbs and cover with a towel.

Steam for 10-15 minutes.

*Where to Find Ingredients:* Lemon verbena and thyme can be found in most health food stores, online herbal shops, or farmers' markets.

**Lavender & Thyme Toner**

This toner is excellent for calming the skin and reducing redness and irritation. The lavender soothes, while the thyme helps to clear up acne.

*Ingredients*

- 1 tablespoon dried lavender flowers
- 1 tablespoon dried thyme
- 1 cup distilled water

*Instructions*

Boil the distilled water and pour it over the dried lavender and thyme.

Let it steep for about 10 minutes.

Strain the herbs and transfer the liquid to a glass jar.

Use a cotton pad to apply the toner to your face after cleansing.

*Where to Find Ingredients:* Both lavender and thyme are widely available in herb shops, health food stores, and online.

**Apple Cider Vinegar & Rose Water Toner**

Apple cider vinegar is a natural astringent that helps balance skin's pH and reduces oil, while rose water soothes and hydrates. This toner is excellent for oily or acne-prone skin.

*Ingredients*

- 2 tablespoons apple cider vinegar
- 2 tablespoons rose water
- 1 cup distilled water

*Instructions*

Combine the apple cider vinegar, rose water, and distilled water in a glass jar.

Shake well before each use.

Apply with a cotton pad to tone the skin after cleansing.

*Where to Find Ingredients:* Apple cider vinegar, rose water, and distilled water can be found at most supermarkets, health food stores, or online.

## ANTI-AGING HERB PROFILES & RECIPES

### Gotu Kola

*Overview:* Gotu Kola is an herb known for its ability to stimulate collagen production and improve the elasticity of the skin.

*Key Benefits*

- Stimulates collagen production.
- Firms and tightens the skin.
- Reduces the appearance of scars.

*Where to Find:* Gotu Kola is available in dried or powdered form at health food stores or online.

### Gotu Kola Firming Serum

2 tablespoons gotu kola powder

1 tablespoon rosehip oil

5 drops lavender essential oil

Mix all ingredients into a serum and apply it nightly to reduce wrinkles and promote firm skin.

### Turmeric

*Overview:* Turmeric is a powerful anti-inflammatory and antioxidant herb that has long been used for its skin benefits, especially in slowing the effects of aging. It helps reduce the appearance of dark spots, wrinkles, and fine lines.

*Key Benefits*

- Brightens complexion.
- Reduces inflammation.
- Prevents the breakdown of collagen.

*Where to Find:* Turmeric powder can be found in any spice section of a grocery store or health food store. Turmeric essential oil and fresh turmeric root are also available online or at specialty stores.

**Anti-Aging Recipe: Turmeric & Yogurt Mask**

- 1 teaspoon turmeric powder
- 2 tablespoons plain yogurt
- 1 teaspoon honey

*Instructions*

Mix all ingredients together in a bowl.

Apply the mask evenly to your face and leave it on for 15 minutes.

Rinse with warm water, followed by cool water to close pores.

**Frankincense**

**Overview:** Frankincense is known for its anti-aging properties. It promotes skin regeneration, helps smooth wrinkles, and reduces the appearance of scars, making it a key herb in any anti-aging skincare routine.

**Key Benefits:**

- Improves skin elasticity.
- Reduces fine lines and wrinkles.
- Increases skin's tone and texture.

**Where to Find:** Frankincense essential oil is widely available at health food stores, aromatherapy stores, and online.

**Anti-Aging Recipe: Frankincense & Jojoba Oil Serum**

- 4 drops frankincense essential oil
- 1 tablespoon jojoba oil
- 1 tablespoon rosehip oil

*Instructions*

Mix the essential oils and oils in a small glass bottle.

Apply a few drops to your face at night before bed for smoother, firmer skin.

**Rosehip Oil**

*Overview:* Rosehip oil is rich in essential fatty acids and antioxidants, making it one of the best natural oils for reducing the signs of aging. It helps to boost collagen production and repair damaged skin.

*Key Benefits*

- Reduces the appearance of scars and stretch marks.
- Improves skin texture and tone.
- Helps regenerate skin cells.

*Where to Find:* Rosehip oil is available at most health food stores and online, typically in organic or cold-pressed forms.

**Anti-Aging Recipe: Rosehip Oil & Lavender Moisturizer**

- 2 tablespoons rosehip oil
- 3 drops lavender essential oil
- 1 tablespoon coconut oil

*Instructions*

Mix all ingredients in a small bowl.

Apply to your face after cleansing and toning, preferably before bed.

# CHAPTER 12
# LIP CARE

## HERBS FOR LIP HEALTH

Our lips are among the most delicate parts of our body. Unlike the rest of our skin, lips lack oil glands, which makes them particularly prone to dryness and damage. Whether you're dealing with chapped lips, cold sores, or other common issues, herbal remedies can provide natural, effective, and gentle solutions to restore and maintain lip health.

Lips can become chapped or damaged due to environmental factors such as harsh weather, dehydration, or exposure to irritants. Cold sores, on the other hand, are caused by the herpes simplex virus (HSV-1) and often flare up during times of stress or when the immune system is weakened. In this chapter, we will explore the best herbs for lip health, provide recipes for care, and discuss natural solutions for these common ailments.

**Why Do We Get Chapped Lips?**

Understanding the root causes of chapped lips is key to preventing and treating this common problem. Some of the most common reasons for chapped lips include:

- **Dehydration**: Lips are one of the first areas to show signs of dehydration. Without adequate water intake, the skin on your lips can quickly dry out.
- **Weather**: Cold, dry air in the winter or excessive heat and sun exposure in the summer can strip moisture from your lips.
- **Licking Your Lips**: While it may seem like a quick fix, licking your lips can actually worsen dryness. Saliva evaporates quickly, leaving lips drier than before.
- **Vitamin Deficiencies**: A lack of certain vitamins, particularly B vitamins, can contribute to dry, cracked lips.
- **Allergic Reactions**: Some lip products contain irritants or allergens that can cause dryness or peeling.
- **Medical Conditions**: Conditions like cheilitis or certain medications can also lead to chronic lip dryness.

Herbal remedies can help address these causes by nourishing the skin, providing hydration, and creating a protective barrier to lock in moisture.

## NATURAL REMEDIES FOR CHAPPED LIPS

### Coconut and Calendula Lip Balm

Calendula, known for its healing and anti-inflammatory properties, is an excellent herb for soothing and repairing dry lips. Combined with coconut oil, it provides deep hydration.

*Ingredients*

- 1 tablespoon dried calendula flowers
- ½ cup coconut oil
- 1 tablespoon beeswax (optional for a firmer balm)
- 3-4 drops of essential oil (such as lavender or peppermint, optional)

*Instructions*

Infuse the coconut oil with calendula by gently heating the oil and flowers in a double boiler for 30 minutes.

Strain the mixture to remove the flowers.

Melt the beeswax (if using) and stir it into the infused oil.

Add essential oils for fragrance and additional benefits.

Pour into small containers and let it cool before use.

*Where to Find Ingredients:* Dried calendula flowers can be found in herbal shops, health food stores, or online. Coconut oil and beeswax are available in most grocery stores or natural food markets. Essential oils can be found online or in specialty aromatherapy shops.

**Honey and Aloe Vera Lip Mask**

Honey is a natural humectant, which means it attracts and retains moisture, while aloe vera soothes irritation and promotes healing.

*Ingredients*

- 1 teaspoon raw honey
- 1 teaspoon fresh aloe vera gel

*Instructions*

Mix the honey and aloe vera gel until well combined.

Apply a thin layer to your lips and leave it on for 15-20 minutes.

Rinse off with lukewarm water and apply a natural lip balm to seal in moisture.

*Where to Find Ingredients:* Raw honey is available at grocery stores or farmers' markets. Fresh aloe vera gel can be extracted directly from the plant, which is often sold at garden centers, or purchased in bottled form from health food stores.

## UNDERSTANDING AND TREATING COLD SORES

Cold sores are caused by the herpes simplex virus and are often triggered by stress, illness, or sun exposure. While there is no cure for the virus, certain herbs can help speed up healing and reduce the frequency of outbreaks.

### Antiviral Herbs for Cold Sores

**Lemon Balm (*Melissa officinalis*)** Lemon balm is a powerful antiviral herb that has been shown to reduce the duration and severity of cold sores. It can be used topically or taken as a tea to support the immune system.

### Lemon Balm Cold Sore Ointment

*Ingredients*

- 2 tablespoons dried lemon balm leaves
- ¼ cup olive oil
- 1 tablespoon beeswax

*Instructions*

Infuse the olive oil with lemon balm by heating gently in a double boiler for 30 minutes.

Strain the mixture and return it to the double boiler.

Add beeswax and stir until melted.

Pour into a small jar and let it cool. Apply to cold sores 2-3 times daily.

*Where to Find Ingredients:* Dried lemon balm leaves can be purchased from herbal shops or online retailers. Olive oil and beeswax are available at grocery stores or natural food markets.

**Licorice Root (*Glycyrrhiza glabra*)** Licorice root contains glycyrrhizin, which has antiviral properties and can help inhibit the herpes virus.

**Licorice Root Paste**

*Ingredients*

- 1 teaspoon licorice root powder
- 2 teaspoons coconut oil or water

*Instructions*

Mix the licorice root powder with coconut oil or water to form a paste.

Apply directly to the cold sore and leave it on for 10-15 minutes.

Rinse off and repeat 2-3 times daily.

*Where to Find Ingredients:* Licorice root powder can be found in herbal stores or online. Coconut oil is widely available in grocery and natural food stores.

**Echinacea** Echinacea boosts the immune system, helping the body fight off infections and reduce the likelihood of cold sore outbreaks. Drink echinacea tea regularly during periods of stress or illness to keep your immune system strong.

**Echinacea Immune-Boosting Tea**

*Ingredients*

- 1 tablespoon dried echinacea
- 1 teaspoon dried peppermint (optional for flavor)
- 1 cup boiling water

*Instructions*

Steep the herbs in boiling water for 10 minutes.

Strain and enjoy up to two cups daily.

*Where to Find Ingredients:* Dried echinacea and peppermint are available at herbal shops, health food stores, or online retailers.

## TIPS FOR PREVENTING LIP AILMENTS

- **Stay Hydrated**: Drink plenty of water to keep your lips and skin hydrated.
- **Use SPF Protection**: Protect your lips from sun damage with a lip balm that contains SPF.
- **Avoid Triggers**: Identify and avoid triggers for cold sores, such as excessive sun exposure or high-stress situations.
- **Boost Your Diet**: Incorporate foods rich in vitamins B, C, and E to support overall lip health.
- **Choose Natural Lip Products**: Avoid lip products with synthetic fragrances or allergens that can irritate sensitive skin.

## ADVANCED HERBAL LIP TREATMENTS

**Chamomile and Rosehip Lip Serum**

Chamomile soothes irritation, while rosehip oil provides deep hydration and helps repair damaged skin.

*Ingredients*

- 1 teaspoon dried chamomile flowers
- 1 tablespoon rosehip oil
- 1 teaspoon jojoba oil

*Instructions*

Infuse the chamomile flowers in rosehip oil by heating gently for 30 minutes.

Strain and combine with jojoba oil.

Store in a roller bottle or small jar. Apply to lips morning and night.

*Where to Find Ingredients:* Dried chamomile flowers can be found in herbal stores or online. Rosehip oil and jojoba oil are available at health food stores or specialty skincare retailers.

# CHAPTER 13
# SKIN CARE

**Understanding Aging Skin**

Our skin evolves as we age, and these changes are a natural part of life. Aging skin becomes thinner, less elastic, and drier, making it more prone to wrinkles, fine lines, and conditions such as crepey skin or tears. Collagen production slows, and the natural fat layer beneath the skin diminishes, leading to less plumpness and increased fragility. Additionally, environmental factors like sun exposure and pollution, combined with lifestyle habits such as diet and hydration, can influence the rate and degree of skin aging.

This chapter explores herbal remedies and natural treatments to nurture aging skin, address common concerns such as calluses, blisters, and warts, and provide effective exfoliating solutions through salt and sugar scrubs. We'll also include practical recipes for various skin treatments, herbal baths, oils, and creams, and guide you on where to find the ingredients for them. Additionally, we will discuss recipes suitable for all skin types. From herbal baths to healing creams and oils, these solutions harness the power of nature to promote skin health and vitality.

## SUGAR VS. SALT SCRUBS: A COMPARISON

Exfoliation is essential for maintaining healthy skin by removing dead skin cells and encouraging cell regeneration. Sugar and salt scrubs are two popular options, each with unique benefits.

**Sugar Scrubs**

- **Gentle Exfoliation:** Sugar has smaller, rounder granules, making it less abrasive and suitable for sensitive or delicate skin, such as facial areas.
- **Hydrating Properties:** Sugar is a natural humectant, which helps retain moisture in the skin.
- **Mild AHA Benefits:** Sugar contains glycolic acid, an alpha hydroxy acid (AHA) that promotes skin cell turnover and improves texture.

**Salt Scrubs**

- **Deep Cleansing:** Salt granules are coarser, making them ideal for areas like elbows, knees, and feet where skin is thicker.
- **Mineral-Rich:** Salt is packed with minerals like magnesium, potassium, and calcium, which can nourish the skin and improve circulation.
- **Detoxifying:** Salt scrubs draw out impurities and toxins, making them great for body care.

**Considerations:** While salt scrubs are excellent for tougher skin, they may irritate sensitive or thin skin due to their coarser texture. Sugar scrubs are generally milder and more versatile for all skin types.

## RECIPES FOR SALT AND SUGAR SCRUBS

### Moisturizing Vanilla Sugar Scrub

This gentle sugar scrub exfoliates while moisturizing and nourishing the skin, leaving it soft and smooth.

*Ingredients*

- 1 cup granulated sugar
- ½ cup coconut oil (or almond oil)
- 1 teaspoon vanilla extract

*Instructions*

Melt the coconut oil if solid, then mix with the sugar in a bowl.

Add the vanilla extract and stir until well combined.

Store in a glass jar and use 2-3 times a week for smooth, hydrated skin.

*Where to Find Ingredients:* Granulated sugar is available in any grocery store. Coconut or almond oil can be found at health food stores or online, and vanilla extract is widely available in the baking section of grocery stores.

### Detoxifying Lavender Salt Scrub

This mineral-rich salt scrub soothes the skin and promotes relaxation with the calming scent of lavender.

*Ingredients*

- 1 cup sea salt (or Himalayan salt)
- ½ cup olive oil
- 10-12 drops lavender essential oil

*Instructions*

Combine the sea salt and olive oil in a mixing bowl.

Add the lavender essential oil and stir thoroughly.

Store in an airtight container and use on the body (avoiding the face) once a week.

*Where to Find Ingredients:* Sea salt and olive oil can be purchased at grocery stores. Lavender essential oil is available in aromatherapy shops, health food stores, or online retailers.

## HERBAL BATHS FOR SKIN HEALTH

Herbal baths provide a relaxing and therapeutic way to improve skin health. They hydrate, soothe irritation, and promote healing.

**Chamomile and Oat Soothing Bath**

This bath is ideal for dry, itchy, or sensitive skin.

*Ingredients*

- 1 cup rolled oats (placed in a muslin bag or sock)
- ½ cup dried chamomile flowers
- 10 drops lavender essential oil (optional)

*Instructions*

Fill your bathtub with warm water.

Add the oats and chamomile flowers to the water.

Drip lavender essential oil into the bath if desired.

Soak for 20-30 minutes.

*Where to Find Ingredients:* Rolled oats are available in grocery stores. Chamomile flowers and lavender essential oil can be purchased at herbal shops or online.

**Rose Petal and Calendula Healing Bath**

This bath is excellent for rejuvenating tired, dull skin and promoting healing.

*Ingredients*

- 1 cup dried rose petals
- ½ cup dried calendula flowers
- 1 tablespoon sea salt

*Instructions*

Mix the rose petals, calendula flowers, and sea salt in a bowl.

Add the mixture to a warm bath and soak for 20-30 minutes.

*Where to Find Ingredients:* Dried rose petals and calendula flowers are available at herbal suppliers or online. Sea salt can be found at grocery stores.

## HERBAL OILS AND CREAMS FOR ALL SKIN TYPES

**Calendula-Infused Skin Oil**

This versatile oil hydrates and soothes all skin types.

*Ingredients*

- ½ cup dried calendula flowers
- 1 cup olive oil

*Instructions*

Place the calendula flowers in a clean jar and cover with olive oil.

Seal the jar and let it sit in a warm spot for 4-6 weeks, shaking occasionally.

Strain the oil and store it in a dark glass bottle.

*Where to Find Ingredients:* Calendula flowers can be sourced from herbal shops. Olive oil is available at any grocery store.

**Herbal Skin Healing Cream**

This cream helps repair damaged skin and is suitable for all skin types.

*Ingredients*

- 1 tablespoon dried comfrey leaves
- 1 tablespoon dried plantain leaves
- ½ cup coconut oil
- 1 tablespoon beeswax

*Instructions*

Infuse the comfrey and plantain leaves in coconut oil by gently heating for 30 minutes.

Strain the oil and return it to the double boiler.

Add beeswax and stir until melted.

Pour into a small container and allow to cool before use.

*Where to Find Ingredients:* Comfrey and plantain leaves are available in herbal shops. Coconut oil and beeswax can be found at health food stores or online.

## SOLUTIONS FOR CREPEY SKIN

Crepey skin, characterized by thin, wrinkled, and sagging texture, often appears on areas like the neck, arms, and under the eyes. This condition can result from a combination of aging, dehydration, and sun damage.

**Herbal Remedies for Crepey Skin**

- **Aloe Vera Gel:** Hydrates and tightens the skin while promoting collagen production.
- **Rosehip Oil:** Rich in vitamin A and essential fatty acids, it improves elasticity and reduces wrinkles.
- **Gotu Kola (Centella asiatica):** Stimulates collagen synthesis and repairs skin.

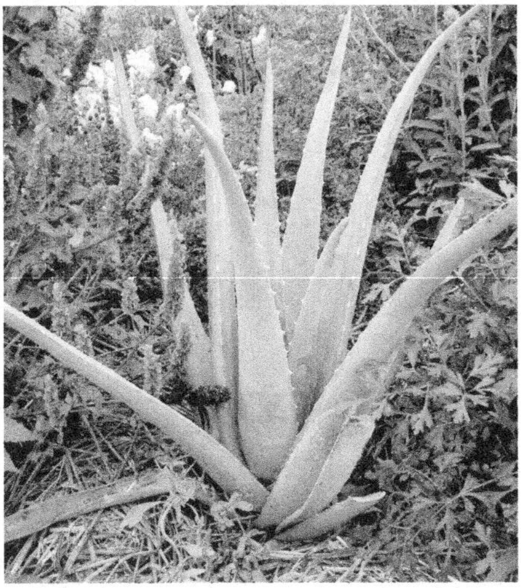

*Aloe*

**Crepey Skin Mask Recipe**

*Ingredients*

- 2 tablespoons aloe vera gel
- 1 teaspoon rosehip oil
- 1 teaspoon gotu kola powder (or tea infusion)

*Instructions*

Mix the aloe vera gel and rosehip oil in a bowl.

Add the gotu kola powder or infusion and blend until smooth.

Apply to the affected areas and leave on for 15-20 minutes.

Rinse with lukewarm water and pat dry.

*Where to Find Ingredients:* Aloe vera gel is sold at health food stores or extracted from fresh aloe plants. Rosehip oil is available in natural skin-care shops or online. Gotu kola powder can be purchased from herbal suppliers or online retailers.

CHAPTER 14

# HANDS AND FEET CARE

## The Importance of Caring for Your Hands and Feet

Our hands and feet endure significant wear and tear daily. From exposure to environmental elements to constant use, they are prone to dryness, calluses, blisters, and other issues. Proper care not only maintains their appearance but also prevents discomfort and long-term problems. In this chapter, we'll explore herbal remedies to address common hand and foot concerns, including herbal soaks, oils, and creams tailored for these hardworking areas. We'll also provide recipes for natural treatments and discuss where to source the ingredients.

**Common Issues of the Hands and Feet**

**Dry Skin:** Often caused by exposure to water, detergents, or cold weather.

**Calluses:** Thickened skin from repeated friction or pressure.

**Cracked Heels:** Caused by dryness and pressure on the feet.

**Blisters:** Fluid-filled pockets resulting from friction or burns.

**Corns:** Painful, hardened areas of skin, often on toes.

**Fungal Infections:** Including athlete's foot, which thrives in moist environments.

Herbal treatments can effectively address these issues by softening, soothing, and protecting the skin.

## HERBAL SOAKS FOR HANDS AND FEET

Herbal soaks are an excellent way to relax, soften the skin, and address specific concerns such as dryness or fungal infections.

**Relaxing Lavender and Epsom Salt Soak**

This soak soothes tired hands and feet while softening the skin.

*Ingredients*

- 1 cup Epsom salt
- 2 tablespoons dried lavender flowers
- 10 drops lavender essential oil
- Warm water (enough to fill a basin)

*Instructions*

Fill a basin with warm water and dissolve the Epsom salt.

Add dried lavender flowers and lavender essential oil.

Soak your hands or feet for 15-20 minutes.

*Where to Find Ingredients:* Epsom salt is available in pharmacies or grocery stores. Dried lavender flowers and essential oils can be purchased from herbal shops or online retailers.

**Antifungal Tea Tree and Rosemary Foot Soak**

This soak helps combat fungal infections and refreshes tired feet.

*Ingredients*

- 1 cup sea salt
- 5 drops tea tree essential oil
- 5 drops rosemary essential oil
- 1 tablespoon dried thyme (optional)

*Instructions*

Combine the sea salt with essential oils in a basin of warm water.

Add dried thyme if desired and stir well.

Soak your feet for 15-20 minutes, ensuring all areas are submerged.

*Where to Find Ingredients:* Sea salt and essential oils are widely available in health food stores or online. Dried thyme can be sourced from grocery stores or herbal shops.

## HERBAL CREAMS AND BALMS FOR HANDS AND FEET

### Calendula and Shea Butter Hand Cream

This rich hand cream soothes dryness and restores hydration.

*Ingredients*

- 1 tablespoon dried calendula flowers
- 1 cup shea butter
- 2 tablespoons almond oil
- 5 drops chamomile essential oil

*Instructions*

Infuse almond oil with calendula flowers by gently heating for 30 minutes.

Strain the oil and mix with melted shea butter.

Add chamomile essential oil and stir well.

Pour into a small jar and let it cool before use.

*Where to Find Ingredients:* Shea butter is available in natural skincare shops or online. Calendula flowers and essential oils can be sourced from herbal suppliers.

**Peppermint Foot Balm**

This cooling balm relieves tired, aching feet and softens cracked heels.

*Ingredients*

- 1 tablespoon dried peppermint leaves
- 1 cup coconut oil
- 1 tablespoon beeswax
- 10 drops peppermint essential oil

*Instructions*

Infuse the coconut oil with peppermint leaves by gently heating for 30 minutes.

Strain the oil and return to the double boiler.

Add beeswax and stir until melted.

Mix in peppermint essential oil and pour into a small container.

Let it cool and solidify before applying to feet.

*Where to Find Ingredients:* Peppermint leaves and essential oil can be purchased from herbal suppliers or online. Beeswax and coconut oil are available in health food stores.

## REMEDIES FOR SPECIFIC HAND AND FOOT ISSUES

### Caring for Calluses, Corns and Blisters

Calluses form due to repeated friction or pressure, often on hands and feet. Soften and remove them with herbal soaks and scrubs.

### Callus-Softening Treatment

*Ingredients*

- 2 tablespoons baking soda
- 1 cup warm water
- 1 tablespoon olive oil

*Instructions*

Dissolve baking soda in warm water.

Soak hands or feet for 15 minutes.

Massage olive oil into the callus and gently exfoliate with a pumice stone.

*Where to Find Ingredients:* Baking soda and olive oil are readily available in grocery stores.

### Blister Healing Salve

*Ingredients*

- 1 tablespoon dried chamomile flowers
- 1 tablespoon dried calendula flowers
- ½ cup olive oil
- 1 tablespoon beeswax

*Instructions*

Infuse olive oil with chamomile and calendula flowers by heating gently for 30 minutes.

Strain the oil and return it to the double boiler.

Add beeswax and stir until melted.

Pour into a container and let cool before applying to blisters.

*Where to Find Ingredients:* Chamomile and calendula flowers can be purchased from herbal shops or online. Olive oil and beeswax are available at grocery stores or natural food markets.

**Fungal Treatment for Athlete's Foot**

*Ingredients*

- 2 tablespoons apple cider vinegar
- 5 drops tea tree essential oil
- 1 cup warm water

*Instructions*

Combine all ingredients in a basin.

Soak feet for 10-15 minutes daily until symptoms improve.

*Where to Find Ingredients:* Apple cider vinegar and tea tree essential oil are available at health food stores or online.

CHAPTER 15

# HOW TO GROW YOUR OWN HERBAL GARDEN

Growing your own herbal garden is a rewarding way to ensure a steady supply of fresh, organic herbs for your remedies. Whether you have a sprawling backyard or a small windowsill, cultivating herbs at home is a simple and sustainable practice that connects you to nature while enhancing your wellness journey. This chapter provides guidance on the best herbs to grow, tips for planting and harvesting, and how to create your own remedies using homegrown herbs.

**Why Grow Your Own Herbal Garden?**

Creating your own herbal garden not only saves money but also ensures you have access to fresh, organic herbs free from harmful chemicals. It allows you to nurture plants that cater to your specific health and wellness needs while connecting with the therapeutic benefits of gardening itself. Research shows that tending to plants can reduce stress, boost mood, and provide a sense of accomplishment. By growing herbs at home, you can develop a sustainable source of ingredients for teas, tinctures, balms, and culinary uses.

## BEST HERBS TO GROW AT HOME

These herbs are versatile, easy to grow, and highly beneficial for culinary and medicinal purposes.

**Basil**

- **Uses:** Supports digestion, reduces inflammation, and enhances immunity.
- **Growing Tips:** Prefers warm, sunny spots with well-draining soil. Water regularly but avoid overwatering.
- **Where to Find Seeds:** Available at garden centers or online seed suppliers.

**Mint**

- **Uses:** Eases digestion, soothes headaches, and freshens breath.
- **Growing Tips:** Thrives in partial shade and moist soil. Grow in containers to prevent spreading.
- **Where to Find Seeds or Plants:** Garden stores, farmers' markets, or online.

**Lavender**

- **Uses:** Promotes relaxation, improves sleep, and supports skin health.
- **Growing Tips:** Needs full sun and well-draining soil. Prune regularly to encourage growth.
- **Where to Find Seeds or Plants:** Nurseries or online herbal suppliers.

**Thyme**

- **Uses:** Antibacterial properties support respiratory health and wound healing.

- **Growing Tips:** Grows well in sunny areas with sandy soil. Avoid overwatering.
- **Where to Find Seeds or Plants:** Garden centers, online stores, or farmers' markets.

**Chamomile**

- **Uses:** Soothes stress, aids sleep, and supports digestion.
- **Growing Tips:** Prefers sunny locations and well-drained soil. Harvest flowers when fully open.
- **Where to Find Seeds:** Garden stores or reputable online seed suppliers.

**Parsley**

- **Uses:** High in vitamins A, C, and K; supports bone health and immunity.
- **Growing Tips:** Grows best in moist, well-draining soil with partial sunlight.
- **Where to Find Seeds:** Available in grocery stores or online seed retailers.

**Lemon Balm**

- **Uses:** Reduces anxiety, promotes sleep, and supports digestion.
- **Growing Tips:** Thrives in partial shade and rich, well-drained soil.
- **Where to Find Seeds or Plants:** Online herbal suppliers or nurseries.

**Echinacea**

- **Uses:** Boosts immunity and supports respiratory health.
- **Growing Tips:** Needs full sun and well-drained soil. Deadhead flowers to prolong blooming.

- **Where to Find Seeds:** Garden centers or online seed suppliers.

**Rosemary**

- **Uses:** Improves memory, supports digestion, and enhances circulation.
- **Growing Tips:** Requires full sun and well-drained soil. Water sparingly.
- **Where to Find Seeds or Plants:** Nurseries, farmers' markets, or online.

**Dill**

- **Uses:** Supports digestion and enhances the flavor of culinary dishes.
- **Growing Tips:** Prefers full sun and well-drained soil. Harvest leaves and seeds as needed.
- **Where to Find Seeds:** Grocery stores or online seed retailers.

## PLANTING AND HARVESTING TIPS

### Choose the Right Location

- Most herbs thrive in areas with plenty of sunlight. Ensure your garden gets at least 6-8 hours of sunlight daily.
- For indoor gardens, place pots near south-facing windows.

### Prepare the Soil

- Use well-draining soil enriched with organic compost.
- Test soil pH to ensure it's neutral to slightly alkaline (6.0-7.5).

**Watering Guidelines**

- Avoid overwatering, as most herbs prefer soil that is slightly dry between watering.
- Water in the morning to prevent fungal growth.

**Harvest Regularly**

- Pick leaves in the morning when essential oils are most concentrated.
- Use sharp scissors or pruners to avoid damaging the plants.

**Pest Control**

- Use natural pest repellents like neem oil or companion planting (e.g., marigolds to deter aphids).

**Container Gardening Tips**

- Choose pots with good drainage holes.
- Use lightweight potting soil and rotate containers regularly to ensure even sun exposure.

**Seasonal Care**

- For perennials like rosemary and thyme, provide frost protection during winter months.
- Rotate annual herbs like basil and cilantro to prevent soil nutrient depletion.

## DIY HERBAL REMEDIES FROM YOUR GARDEN

**Lavender Sleep Sachets**

*Ingredients*

- 1 cup dried lavender flowers
- Small fabric bags

*Instructions*

1. Fill each fabric bag with dried lavender flowers.
2. Tie the bags securely and place them under your pillow for better sleep.

*Where to Find Ingredients:* Grow lavender at home or purchase dried lavender online.

**Mint-Infused Water**

*Ingredients*

- 1/4 cup fresh mint leaves
- 1 liter of water

*Instructions*

1. Add fresh mint leaves to a pitcher of water.
2. Let it infuse for at least 2 hours in the refrigerator.
3. Enjoy as a refreshing and digestive aid.

*Where to Find Ingredients:* Fresh mint can be grown at home or purchased at grocery stores.

**Thyme and Honey Cough Syrup**

*Ingredients*

- 1/2 cup fresh thyme leaves
- 1 cup raw honey

*Instructions*

1. Gently heat honey and thyme in a saucepan for 10 minutes.
2. Strain and store in a sterilized jar.
3. Take 1 teaspoon as needed to soothe coughs.

*Where to Find Ingredients:* Fresh thyme is available at grocery stores or from your garden.

**Chamomile Facial Steam**

*Ingredients*

- 1/4 cup dried chamomile flowers
- 4 cups boiling water

*Instructions*

Add chamomile flowers to a bowl and pour boiling water over them.

Cover your head with a towel and lean over the bowl for 5-10 minutes.

Rinse your face with cool water.

*Where to Find Ingredients:* Dried chamomile flowers can be purchased online or grown at home.

**Lemon Balm Tincture**

*Ingredients*

- 1 cup fresh lemon balm leaves
- 2 cups high-proof alcohol (like vodka)

*Instructions*

Place lemon balm leaves in a sterilized jar.

Cover with alcohol and seal tightly.

Store in a dark, cool place for 4-6 weeks, shaking occasionally.

Strain and store in a dropper bottle. Use 1-2 droppers daily for stress relief.

*Where to Find Ingredients:* Grow lemon balm at home or purchase fresh leaves from farmers' markets.

# CONCLUSION

Holistic wellness is a journey, not a destination. It encompasses nurturing the mind, body, and spirit through natural and balanced approaches that prioritize harmony with nature. By embracing the power of herbal remedies, you've taken an essential step toward reclaiming control of your health in a way that is sustainable, gentle, and effective. The knowledge shared throughout this book is rooted in centuries of tradition, coupled with modern insights, to help you unlock the profound benefits of herbs and natural healing practices.

Through consistent application of these remedies, you'll discover how small, intentional changes—whether it's brewing a calming tea, incorporating fresh herbs into your diet, or creating your own tinctures—can lead to transformative results. Remember, the goal isn't perfection but progress toward a lifestyle that honors your unique needs and the wisdom of the natural world.

The world of herbal remedies is vast and filled with endless opportunities to learn and grow. As you've seen, herbs are not merely tools for addressing ailments—they are gateways to a deeper connection with nature and yourself. This book is just the beginning of your journey. Continue to explore, experiment, and expand your knowledge of herbs and their applications. Try cultivating new plants in your garden, creating personalized blends, or diving deeper into the history and cultural significance of herbal medicine.

Keep in mind that holistic wellness thrives on curiosity and adaptability. As you encounter new challenges in life, turn to the principles of balance and natural healing to guide you. Trust your intuition and let the wisdom of plants inspire your journey toward better health and well-being.

As you close this book, take pride in the knowledge you've gained and the steps you've taken toward holistic wellness. May your path be one of health, harmony, and abundant growth.

# INDEX

**P**



**R**



**S**



**T**



**V**



**W**

# PHOTO CREDITS

https://commons.wikimedia.org/wiki/File:Vue_du_batiment_principal_de_l%27herboristerie_La_F%C3%A9e_des_bois_%C3%A0_-Clarendon_(Qu%C3%A9bec)-2024-05-12.jpg

https://commons.wikimedia.org/wiki/File:Herbal_medicine_platter.jpg

https://commons.wikimedia.org/wiki/File:Washing_hands_with_soap_(2).jpg

https://commons.wikimedia.org/wiki/File:Lavandula_latifolia_plant_(21).jpg

https://commons.wikimedia.org/wiki/File:Tea_herbal.jpg

https://commons.wikimedia.org/wiki/File:Allium_sativum._Restra_de_allos_de_Oroso-_Galiza.jpg

https://commons.wikimedia.org/wiki/File:Teatreeoil.jpg

https://commons.wikimedia.org/wiki/File:New_olive_oil,_just_pressed.jpg

https://commons.wikimedia.org/wiki/File:Peppermint20020515.jpg

https://commons.wikimedia.org/wiki/File:Dandelion_Flower_close_up.jpg

https://commons.wikimedia.org/wiki/File:Sweet_Basil_(Ocimum_basilicum).jpg

https://commons.wikimedia.org/wiki/File:Eucalyptus_robusta_-_flowers.jpg

https://commons.wikimedia.org/wiki/File:Rose_hip_in_Rind_village.jpg

https://commons.wikimedia.org/wiki/File:Lemon.jpg

https://commons.wikimedia.org/wiki/File:
Rosmarinus_officinalis_(Lamiaceae).jpg

https://commons.wikimedia.org/wiki/File:Humulus_lupulus_with_fly.jpg

https://commons.wikimedi-
a.org/wiki/File:Proven%C3%A7al_herbs,_Saint-Paul_de_Vence.JPG

https://commons.wikimedia.org/wiki/File:Evening_Primrose_-_geo
graph.org.uk_-_3613401.jpg

https://commons.wikimedia.org/wiki/File:
Turmeric_Root_and_Turmeric_Powder.jpg

https://commons.wikimedia.org/wiki/File:-2019-10-

https://commons.wikimedia.org/wiki/File:Yoghurt_and_spoon.jpg

https://commons.wikimedia.org/wiki/File:
Cinnamomum_verum_spices.jpg

https://commons.wikimedia.org/wiki/File:Ringelblume_(Calendula_of-
ficinalis)_Bl%C3%BCte_focus_stack-20220619-RM-165610.jpg

https://commons.wikimedia.org/wiki/File:Aloe_vera_2.jpg

https://vitalityhealingnd.com/blog/podcast-2

Made in the USA
Las Vegas, NV
26 October 2026

56561852R10098